Get Through
MRCOG Part 1

About the Series

Our bestselling *Get Through* series guides medical postgraduates through the many exams they will need to pass throughout their career, whatever their specialty. Each title is written by authors with recent first-hand experience of the exam, overseen and edited by experts in the field to ensure each question or scenario closely matches the latest examining board guidelines. Detailed explanations and background knowledge provide all you need to know to get through your postgraduate medical examination.

Get Through MRCOG Part 1, Second Edition
Rekha Wuntakal, Ziena Abdullah, and Tony Hollingworth

Get Through MRCOG Part 2: EMQs
Kalaivani Ramalingam, Latha Mageswari Palanivelu, Lakshmi Thirumalaikumar

Get Through MRCOG Part 3: Clinical Assessment, Second Edition
T Justin Clark, Arri Coomarasamy, Justin Chu and Paul Smith

Get Through MRCOG Part 2: SBAs
Rekha Wuntakal, Madhavi Kalindindi and Tony Hollingworth

Get Through Final FRCR 2A: SBAs
Teck Yew Chin, Susan Cheng Shelmerdine, Akash Ganguly and Chinedum Anoksike

Get Through MRCPsych Paper A1
Mock Examination Papers
Melvyn WB Zheng, Cyrus SH Ho, Roger Ho, Ian H Treasaden and Basant K Puri

Get Through MRCPsych CASC
Melvyn WB Zheng, Cyrus SH Ho, Roger Ho, Ian H Treasaden and Basant K Puri

Get Through MRCS Part A: SBAs
Nikhil Pawa, Paul Cathcart and Howard Tribe

Get Through DRCOG: SBAs, EMQs and MCQs
Rekha Wuntakal, Madhavi Kalidindi and Tony Hollingworth

For more information about this series, please visit: *https://www.crcpress.com/ Get-Through/book-series/CRCGETTHROUG*

Get Through MRCOG Part 1

Second Edition

Rekha Wuntakal, MBBS, MRCOG, MD, DNB, DFFP

Subspecialist in Gynaecological Oncology
Consultant in Gynaecology and Gynaecological Oncology
Barking, Havering and Redbridge NHS University Hospitals
Romford, UK

Ziena Abdullah, MBBS, BSc, MRCOG, PGCert (Clinical Leadership)

Locum Consultant in Obstetrics and Gynaecology
Barking, Havering and Redbridge NHS University Hospitals
Romford, UK

Tony Hollingworth, MB ChB, MBA, PhD, FRCS(Ed), FRCOG

Gynaecologist
Whipps Cross University Hospital/Barts Health NHS Trust
and Part-time Clinical Research Fellow
Wolfson Institute for Preventive Medicine
Queen Mary University of London
London, UK

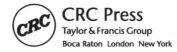

CRC Press
Taylor & Francis Group
Boca Raton London New York

CRC Press is an imprint of the
Taylor & Francis Group, an **informa** business

Second edition published 2020
by CRC Press
6000 Broken Sound Parkway NW, Suite 300, Boca Raton, FL 33487-2742

and by CRC Press
2 Park Square, Milton Park, Abingdon, Oxon, OX14 4RN

© 2021 Taylor & Francis Group, LLC

First edition published by CRC Press, 2010

CRC Press is an imprint of Taylor & Francis Group, LLC

ISBN: 978-0-367-13970-4 (hbk)
ISBN: 978-0-367-13962-9 (pbk)
ISBN: 978-0-429-02947-9 (ebk)

Typeset in Minion
by Lumina Datamatics Limited

CONTENTS

Dedicated to my mum Akkamahadevi, sister Neelu, brothers
Sateesh, Nagaraj and Manjunath and my teachers and students
who have encouraged and inspired me to teach and learn.

Rekha Wuntakal

Dedicated to my mother Sajida, father Abdul-Razaq, husband
Hassan, sister Ayat, my brothers, my late aunty Badriyya, and
the wonderful children in our lives Eisa, Musa and Meriem.

Ziena Abdullah

AUTHORS

Rekha Wuntakal is actively involved in education and training. She had taken time out during training to be an educational fellow to teach medical students from Queen Mary University and Royal London Medical School and has been undergraduate examiner for QMUL. As a consultant, she is actively involved in undergraduate and postgraduate teaching. She has published a number of MRCOG and DRCOG preparation books and is actively involved in teaching on MRCOG Part 1, Part 2 and Part 3 courses.

Ziena Abdullah qualified from Barts and The London Medical School in 2007 with an interacted BSc in Experimental Pathology. She entered the training programme in 2009 and took time out from programme to become a Darzi Fellow and hence to achieve a Postgraduate Certificate in Clinical Leadership. She is currently completing a Postgraduate Certificate in Higher Education from Queen Mary University and has a certificate in gynaecology scanning. She has written numerous papers and books and runs courses for the MRCOG Part 2 and takes part in Part 3 courses.

Tony Hollingworth has experience as an undergraduate and postgraduate examiner both within the UK and overseas. Former Chair of the RCOG OSCE (Part 2) Committee, as well as a member of the RCOG Examinations and Part 3 Committees, he has published a number of MRCOG preparation books. He is currently a member of the Council of the British Society for the Study of Vulval Disease.

LIST OF ABBREVIATIONS

ACE	angiotensin-converting enzyme
ACTH	adrenocorticotropic hormone
ADP	adenosine diphosphate
AFP	alpha-fetoprotein
ANA	antinuclear antibody
APH	antepartum haemorrhage
APS	antiphospholipid antibody syndrome
APTT	activated partial thromboplastin time
ATP	adenosine triphosphate
BCG	Bacillus Calmette–Guérin
BCKDH	branched chain alpha-ketoacid-dehydrogenase complex
BMI	body mass index
C1	complement 1
C2	complement 2
C3	complement 3
CAH	congenital adrenal hyperplasia
cAMP	adenosine cyclic monophosphate
CEMACH	Confidential Enquiries into Maternal Deaths
cGMP	guanosine cyclic monophosphate
CIN	cervical intraepithelial neoplasia
CK	creatine kinase
CMV	cytomegalovirus
CNS	central nervous system
CoA	coenzyme A
COCP	combined oral contraceptive pill
copper IUD	copper intrauterine contraceptive device
CRH	corticotropin-releasing hormone
CTPA	computed tomographic pulmonary angiography
CVS	chorionic villus biopsy
DHEA	dehydroepiandrosterone
DHT	dihydrotestosterone
DIC	disseminated intravascular coagulation
DNA	deoxyribonucleic acid
DOPA	3,4-dihydroxy-phenylalanine
DUB	dysfunctional uterine bleeding
DVT	deep vein thrombosis
E	early
E2	oestrogen 2 (receptor)
EBV	Epstein–Barr virus
ECG	electrocardiograph
ELISA	enzyme-linked immunosorbent assay
ER	endoplasmic reticulum
FBC	full blood count
FDA	Food and Drug Administration
FDPs	fibrin degradation products
FISH	fluorescence in situ hybridization
FSH	follicle-stimulating hormone
G1PUT	galactose-1-phosphate uridyl transferase
G6PD	glucose-6-phosphate dehydrogenase deficiency

GABA	gamma-aminobutyric acid	MHC	major histocompatibility complex
GFR	glomerular filtration rate	MI	mechanical index
GI	gastrointestinal	MMR	measles, mumps and rubella
GnRH	gonadotropin-releasing hormone	MRSA	methicillin-resistant *Staphylococcus aureus*
GTP	guanosine triphosphate	NAD	nicotinamide adenine dinucleotide
GUM	genitourinary medicine		
H_2O_2	hydrogen peroxide	NHS	National Health Service
HbA	haemoglobin A	NICE	National Institute for Health and Clinical Excellence
HbC	haemoglobin C		
HbSS	haemoglobin SS	NK	natural killer
HBV	hepatitis B virus	NPV	negative predictive value
hCG	human chorionic gonadotropin	OHSS	ovarian hyperstimulation syndrome
HDL	high-density lipoprotein	OR	odds ratio
HELLP	haemolysis, elevated liver enzymes and low platelets	ORF	open reading frame
		PAPP-A	pregnancy-associated plasma protein A
HGPRT	hypoxanthine–guanine phosphoribosyl transferase	PCOS	polycystic ovarian syndrome
		PCR	polymerase chain reaction
HIV	human immunodeficiency virus	PE	pulmonary embolism
		PGE2	prostaglandin E2
HMB	heavy menstrual bleeding	PGG2	prostaglandin G2
HMG-CoA	hydroxymethylglutaryl coenzyme A	PGH2	prostaglandin H2
		PID	pelvic inflammatory disease
hPL	human placental lactogen	PPH	postpartum haemorrhage
HPV	human papillomavirus	PPV	positive predictive value
HSV	herpes simplex virus	PT	prothrombin time
HTLV	human T-cell lymphoma virus	RBC	red blood cell
		RDS	respiratory distress syndrome
IgG	immunoglobulin G		
IL IgM	interleukin immunoglobulin M	RNA	ribonucleic acid
		RR	relative risk
IUGR	intrauterine growth retardation	SERM	selective oestrogen receptor modulator
IUS	intrauterine system	SHBG	sex hormone-binding globulin
KOH	potassium hydroxide		
L	late	SLE	systemic lupus erythematosus
LBC	liquid-based cytology		
LDL	low-density lipoprotein	SRY	gene sex-determining region on Y chromosome
LH	luteinizing hormone		
LLETZ	large loop excision of transformation zone	TB	tuberculosis
		TCA	tricarboxylic acid cycle
LPS	lipopolysaccharide	TI	thermal index
MAO	monoamine oxidase	TIB	bone thermal index

TIBC	total iron-binding capacity	**uE3**	urinary estriol
TIS	soft tissue thermal index	**V/Q**	ventilation–perfusion ratio
TNF-α	tumour necrosis factor alpha	**VLDL**	very-low-density lipoprotein
TRH	thyroid hormone- or thyrotropin-releasing hormone	**VRE**	vancomycin-resistant enterococcus
TSH	thyroid-stimulating hormone	**VZ**	varicella zoster
TT	thrombin time	**WBC**	white blood cell count
TZ	transformation zone	**WHO**	World Health Organization

INTRODUCTION

The Membership of the Royal College of Obstetricians and Gynaecologists (MRCOG) examination can be considered the most important international postgraduate examination in obstetrics and gynaecology. It is divided into three parts. Part 1 of the MRCOG examines candidates' knowledge of the basic and applied sciences relevant to the clinical practice of obstetrics and gynaecology. The new curriculum is set out in a series of modules (Knowledge Areas) which outlines knowledge requirements and capabilities in practice to be achieved in relevant training period. One has to pass the MRCOG part 1 exam in order to progress from ST2 to ST3 in O&G training. This information can be easily accessed through the RCOG website, available at:

- https://www.rcog.org.uk/en/careers-training/specialty-training-curriculum/core-curriculum/knowledge-requirements/
- https://www.rcog.org.uk/en/careers-training/specialty-training-curriculum/core-curriculum/current/

Format and syllabus of the part 1 MRCOG exam

The part 1 MRCOG is a written exam. It consists of two papers, each containing 100 single best answer (SBA) questions. Each paper counts for 50% of the overall mark and each question is worth 1 mark. Thus, the result is based on the combined marks of the two papers. Each paper lasts 2.5 hours and there is a lunch break in between.

Each question has a lead-in question followed by five options. The options tend to be in alphabetical or numerical order. The concept is that you select the single answer that fits best with the question stem. Even if you feel that there are several correct answers, you are required to pick the most likely option from the list. There is no negative marking, so you are advised to answer every question.

There is no minimum score required for each paper. The result is determined mainly by a candidate's overall combined marks.

The aim of the examination is to assess candidates' understanding of the basic clinical sciences and how they influence and affect clinical practice.

This book sets out SBAs that cover the syllabus of the MRCOG Part 1. The examination will have been blueprinted to ensure an even coverage of the subjects and domains from the new curriculum modules (Knowledge Areas) and syllabus. This book should therefore be used as an adjunct to your revision, and familiarity with the format of SBAs will be important to succeed in the examination. However, this should not be used as a substitute for ensuring adequate preparation of the basic sciences, which will stand one in good stead for clinical practice and the subsequent Part 2 of the MRCOG examination.

Reference material

MRCOG 1 format:

- https://www.rcog.org.uk/en/careers-training/mrcog-exams/part-1-mrcog/format/

MRCOG 1 syllabus:

- https://www.rcog.org.uk/en/careers-training/mrcog-exams/part-1-mrcog/syllabus/

Recommended reading

RCOG online learning resource: StratOG:

- https://elearning.rcog.org.uk/

RCOG green top guidelines and scientific impact papers:

- https://www.rcog.org.uk/guidelines

FSRH guidelines:

- https://www.fsrh.org/standards-and-guidance/
- https://www.fsrh.org/standards-and-guidance/current-clinical-guidance/

NICE guidelines:

- https://www.guidelines.co.uk/nice/2106.bio
- https://www.guidelines.co.uk/searchresults?qkeyword=Obstetrics+
- https://www.guidelines.co.uk/searchresults?qkeyword=Gynaecology+
- https://www.guidelines.co.uk/searchresults?qkeyword=Contraception+

Arulkumaran S, Symonds I, Fowlie A. *Oxford Handbook of Obstetrics and Gynaecology*. New York: Oxford University Press, 2004.

Bennett PN, Brown MJ. *Clinical Pharmacology*, 10th edn. Edinburgh, Scotland: Churchill Livingstone, 2008.

Bhatnagar SM, Kothari ML, Mehta LA. *Essentials of Human Genetics*, 4th edn. Bombay, India: Orient Longman, 1999.

Bland M. *Introduction to Medical Statistics*, 3rd edn. New York: Oxford University Press, 2000.

Chard T, Lilford R. *Basic Sciences for Obstetrics and Gynaecology*, 5th edn. New York: Springer, 2000.

de Swiet M, Chamberlain G, Bennett P. *Basic Science in Obstetrics and Gynaecology: A Textbook for MRCOG Part 1*, 3rd edn. New York: Churchill Livingstone, 2001.

Ganong WF. *Review of Medical Physiology*, 22nd edn. New York: McGraw-Hill, 2005.

Kingston H. *ABC of Clinical Genetics*, 3rd edn. London, UK: Wiley-Blackwell, 2002.

Kumar V, Abbas AK, Fausto N, Mitchell R. *Robbins Basic Pathology*, 8th edn. Philadelphia, PA: Saunders, 2007.

Ledger WL, Murphy MG. *The MRCOG: A Guide to the Examination*, 3rd edn. London, UK: RCOG Press, 2008.

Murray RK, Granner DK, Mayes P, Rodwell V. Harper's illustrated biochemistry, 27th edn. New York: McGraw-Hill, 2006.

RCOG. Past papers – MRCOG Part 1 multiple choice questions, 1997–2001. London, UK: RCOG Press, 2004.

Reid JL, Rubin PC, Walters M. *Lecture Notes: Clinical Pharmacology and Therapeutics*, 7th edn. London, UK: Wiley-Blackwell, 2006.

Sadler TW. *Langman's Medical Embryology*, 11th edn. Philadelphia, PA: Lippincott Williams & Wilkins, 2009.

Sinnatamby CS. *Last's Anatomy: Regional and Applied*, 12th edn. New York: Churchill Livingstone, 2011.

KNOWLEDGE AREA I: CLINICAL SKILLS

QUESTIONS

1. How many appraisals are there in one revalidation cycle?
   a. One
   b. Two
   c. Three
   d. Four
   e. Five

2. You are the senior house officer (SHO) on labour ward, and you have just managed your first major post-partum haemorrhage case. The patient lost 1500 mL of blood and is now well. You want to be assessed on how you managed the case. Which assessment tool would you use?
   a. Case-based discussion
   b. Mini-CEX
   c. Team observation 1
   d. Write an essay
   e. OSAT

3. A model that is used regularly to break bad news is Kaye's 10-point model (1996). Which of the following is not one of the 10 points?
   a. Allow denial
   b. Do not encourage ventilation of feelings at this stage
   c. Give a warning shot
   d. Preparation
   e. What does the woman know?

4. A 14-year-old girl presents to accident and emergency (A&E) department with abdominal pain and dizziness. She is accompanied by her parents. The pregnancy test is positive, and the FAST scan reveals blood in the abdomen. She is becoming tachycardic and hypotensive. The consultant believes she has a ruptured ectopic, and the patient needs to go to theatre for a salpingectomy. She refuses, and her parents do not know that she is sexually active. What is the correct course of action?
   a. Discuss with another consultant
   b. Discuss with the patient's general practitioner (GP)
   c. Proceed to go to theatre and perform a salpingectomy
   d. Respect the patient's decision
   e. Take consent from the parents

5. You are about to teach five medical students how to perform neonatal resuscitation. Which method of teaching would you adopt?
   a. Bedside training
   b. Problem-based learning
   c. Lecture based
   d. Self-directed learning
   e. Simulated training

ANSWERS

1. e. Five

    Revalidation occurs every 5 years and an appraisal occurs every year, hence five appraisals in one revalidation cycle.

    Further reading

    - RCOG online learning resource. StratOG: Appraisal. https://elearning.rcog.org.uk/appraisal/appraisal
    - Fox R, Kane S. Appraisal for postgraduate trainees. *The Obstetrician & Gynaecologist* 2004; 5:7–10.

2. a. Case-based discussion

    A case-based assessment should be undertaken. It will allow the trainee and the assessor to discuss the management of the case, what went well and what can be improved upon. It will allow the trainee to reflect upon and learn from any potential mistakes.

    Further reading

    - RCOG online learning resource. StratOG: Assessment. https://elearning.rcog.org.uk/assessment/assessment
    - RCOG eLearning Workplace Behaviour and Skills tutorial on *Step up*. https://elearning.rcog.org.uk/tutorials/workplace-behaviour-and-skills

3. b. Do not encourage ventilation of feelings at this stage

Kaye's 10-point model for breaking bad news (BBN)	
Kay's model includes the following:	• Preparation • What does he/she know • Is more information wanted? • Give a warning shot • Allow denial • If requested explain • Listen to the concerns • Ventilation of feelings should be encouraged • Always summarize and plan • Further information should be offered

Further reading

- Kaye P. *Breaking Bad News (pocket book): A 10-step Approach.* Northampton, UK: EPL Publications, 1996.
- Buckman R. *Breaking Bad News: A Guide for Health Care Professionals.* Baltimore, MD: Johns Hopkins University Press, 1992.

4. c. Proceed to go to theatre and perform a salpingectomy

In the case of a minor, they can agree to treatment but cannot refuse it if it is believed to be in their best interest.

Further reading

- GMC. 0–18 years: Guidance for all doctors. Sections 30–33.
- Royal College of Obstetricians and Gynaecologists. *Obtaining Valid Consent for Complex Gynaecological Surgery: Clinical Governance Advice No. 6b.* London, UK: RCOG Press, 2010.

5. e. Simulated training

Simulated training will allow each student to see how the resuscitation is performed and then to actually try the resuscitation himself or herself. It creates a scenario as close to real life as possible.

Further reading

- RCOG online learning resource. StratOG. Teaching.
- Duthie SJ, Garden AS. The teacher, the learner and the method. *The Obstetrician & Gynaecologist* 2010; 12:273–280.

KNOWLEDGE AREA 2: TEACHING AND RESEARCH

QUESTIONS

1. Which of the following is the definition of neonatal death rate?
   a. The number of deaths at 0–10 days per 1000 live births
   b. The number of deaths at 0–20 days per 1000 live births
   c. The number of deaths at 0–27 days per 1000 live births
   d. The number of deaths at 0–27 days per 500 live births
   e. The number of deaths at 0–27 days per 10,000 live births

2. Regarding prevalence and incidence, which of the following is false?
   a. Prevalence is a measure of disease occurrence
   b. Incidence is a measure of disease occurrence
   c. Incidence = prevalence × time
   d. Prevalence is total number of cases detected at a particular point of time
   e. Incidence is a measure of new cases over a particular period of time

3. Which of the following is a requirement of a screening test?
   a. The test should have a low sensitivity
   b. The test should have a low specificity
   c. The test does not have to be cost-effective
   d. The test should be safe to apply to some of the population
   e. There should be a latent period in disease progression

4. Regarding relative risk (RR), which of the following statements is true?
   a. It is a measure of association used to interpret cohort study
   b. It is the ratio of the risk in an unexposed group compared with the exposed group
   c. RR = 1 means that there is definite exposure–outcome association
   d. RR of 3 means that there isn't stronger exposure–outcome association
   e. RR < 1 means that the exposure–outcome association is very strong

5. The result of a study of risk factors for caesarean section in obese women showed that spontaneous onset of labour had a relative risk of 0.76, and the use of misoprostol for the induction of labour had a relative risk of 2.8. Which of the following statements is correct with regard to this study?
   a. Spontaneous onset of labour and caesarean section have a very strong association
   b. Spontaneous onset of labour and caesarean section have a moderately strong association
   c. Misoprostol use for induction of labour and caesarean section does not have a strong association
   d. Misoprostol use for induction of labour is protective and not associated with caesarean section
   e. Spontaneous onset of labour is protective against caesarean section, and misoprostol use increases the risk of caesarean section

6. Regarding randomized controlled studies, which of the following statements is false?
   a. They are observational studies
   b. They are the gold standards of clinical research
   c. An intervention under investigation is compared with standard treatment
   d. An intervention under investigation is compared with a placebo
   e. In such studies, patients are allocated in random fashion to the two groups

7. Regarding meta-analysis, which of the following is incorrect?
   a. Amalgamation technique to combine statistical results from similar clinical trials
   b. Involves measures to minimize biases of various kinds
   c. Involves measures to minimize the effects of chance
   d. Patients in one trial are directly compared with those in another trial
   e. Summary statistics are calculated for each trial

8. With regard to hypothesis testing, which of the following is correct?
   a. Null hypothesis specifies a hypothesized real value for a parameter
   b. Type I error occurs when the null hypothesis is not rejected when it is false
   c. Type II error occurs when the null hypothesis is rejected when it is true
   d. The power of the test is the probability of accepting the null hypothesis when it is false
   e. An alternative hypothesis specifies a real value for a parameter which will be considered when the null hypothesis is not rejected

ANSWERS

1. c.   The number of deaths at 0–27 days per 1000 live births

Definitions of death rates after birth of baby	
Early neonatal deaths or death rates	• Are deaths at 0–6 days of life per 1000 live births
Late neonatal deaths or death rates	• Are those deaths occurring between 7 and 27 days of life per 1000 live births
Neonatal deaths or death rates	• Are those deaths occurring between 0 and 27 days of life per 1000 live births
Postneonatal deaths or death rates	• Are those deaths or the number of deaths occurring after >28 days of birth but <1 year per 1000 live births

Further reading

- RCOG Strat OG-Assessment of the newborn and common neonatal problems.
- Mugglestone MA, Murphy MS, Visintin C, Howe DT, Turner MA. Antibiotics for early-onset neonatal infection: A summary of the NICE guideline 2012. *The Obstetrician & Gynaecologist* 2014; 16:87–92.

2. c.   Incidence = prevalence × time

Note

$$Prevalence = incidence \times time$$

Further reading

- RCOG online learning resource: StratOG: Assessing Evidence.

3. e.   There should be a latent period in disease progression
Screening test: Tests (e.g. cervical smear, blood tests, clinical examinations and procedures) that are used to screen healthy people to identify an unrecognized disease or condition. These are not diagnostic tests. The people who are screen positive will need further investigations in order to make a diagnosis and undertake treatment if needed.

Further reading

- RCOG online learning resource: StratOG: Assessing Evidence.
- Royal College of Obstetricians and Gynaecologists. *How Evidence Can Influence Clinical Practice. SAC Opinion Paper 28.* London, UK: RCOG Press, 2011.

4. a. Is a measure of association used to interpret cohort study

   Note

   It is the ratio of the risk in an exposed group to that in the unexposed group. RR = 1 means that there is no exposure–outcome association. RR < 1 means that there is decreased risk or association between exposure and outcome.

   Further reading

   - Joy J, McClure N. The art of reviewing a paper. *The Obstetrician & Gynaecologist* 2014; 16:129–134.
   - RCOG online learning resource: StratOG: Assessing Evidence.

5. e. Spontaneous onset of labour is protective against caesarean section, and misoprostol use increases the risk of caesarean section

   Relative risk and risk ratio definition and interpretation of results

Relative risk (RR): The ratio of probability of outcome in one group of people compared with another group
RR = 1 means no difference in risk between exposure and outcome
RR < 1 means decreased risk between exposure and outcome
RR > 1 means increased risk between exposure and outcome
Risk ratio: The ratio of risk of events/outcome or side effects occurring in exposed or experimental group compared with control group

   Further reading

   - RCOG online learning resource: StratOG: Assessing Evidence.
   - Oxman AD, Cook DJ, Guyatt GH. Users' guides to the medical literature. VI: How to use an overview. *JAMA* 1994; 272:1367–1371 [Abstract]

6. a. They are observational studies
   Randomized controlled studies are a type of parallel study.

Types of studies	
Retrospective studies	A study that involves collecting information about the past. This could be based on patient recall or how well notes are recorded
Cohort studies	A study that identifies a group of people and follows them over a period of time to see how their exposures affect their outcomes
Case-control studies	A study that compares a group of patients who have a specific condition with a group of patients that do not have it, and looks back in time to see how the two groups differ

   (Continued)

Types of studies	
Parallel studies	These are prospective longitudinal studies (these observe a process over a period of time to investigate changes) performed during the later phases of the evaluation of interventions, where the intervention under investigation is directly compared with the standard treatment or placebo
Randomized controlled trials	These are the gold standard of clinical research. These are parallel studies where patients are randomly allocated to intervention and standard treatment or placebo. There can be two or more arms in the study

Note: Randomization is a method based on chance by which study participants are assigned to a treatment group.

Further reading

- RCOG online learning resource: StratOG: Assessing Evidence.
- CEBM. Centre for Evidence Based Medicine.

7. d. Patients in one trial are directly compared with those in another trial
Patients in one trial are not directly compared with those in another trial. Each trial is analysed separately. Summary statistics are added together in the meta-analysis.

Systematic review is a scientific evaluation of several studies conducted on a specific clinical condition. They are mostly conducted on randomized controlled trials but also on other studies depending on the condition being analysed.

Further reading

- RCOG online learning resource: StratOG: Assessing Evidence.
- Joy J, McClure N. The art of reviewing a paper. *The Obstetrician & Gynaecologist* 2014; 16:129–134.

8. a. Null hypothesis specifies a hypothesized real value for a parameter

Statistics and interpretation of results depending on *p*-value	
Null hypothesis	States that no relationship exists between the variables and outcome of the study • Any observed association occurs by chance (presumed answer to any scientific question until proved otherwise)
The *p*-value	• Is used to accept or reject the null hypothesis in a study • Significant results are those unlikely to have occurred by chance, thus rejecting the null hypothesis • Non-significant results are those where a chance occurrence has not been ruled out, thus the null hypothesis has not been disproved • $p < 0.05$ (probability of obtaining a result by chance is $<1{:}20$) is the accepted threshold for a statistical significance or minimum evidence needed to discard the null hypothesis

(Continued)

Statistics and interpretation of results depending on p-value	
Type I error	• Occurs when the null hypothesis is rejected when it is actually true • For example, there is significant difference ($p < 0.05$) between the samples when it is actually not true • An alternative hypothesis specifies a real value for a parameter that will be considered when the null hypothesis is rejected
Type II error	• Occurs when the null hypothesis is not rejected when it is false • For example, failing to find a significant result ($p \leq 0.05$) between the samples when it really exists

Further reading

• RCOG online learning resource: StratOG: Assessing Evidence.
• Royal College of Obstetricians and Gynaecologists. *How Evidence Can Influence Clinical Practice. SAC Opinion Paper 28.* London, UK: RCOG Press, 2011.

QUESTIONS

1. A 25-year-old woman, para 3, attends the gynaecology clinic as she wishes to have laparoscopic sterilization. She wants to know about the failure rate of the procedure. Which of the following options is correct?
   a. 1 in 100 procedures
   b. 1 in 200 procedures
   c. 1 in 600 procedure
   d. 1 in 1000 procedures
   e. 1 in 2000 procedures

2. A 40-year-old woman attends the gynaecology clinic. She wishes to have laparoscopic sterilization and is worried about risks of the procedure.
   Which of the following is not correct regarding the risks of this procedure?
   a. Bladder injury is 1 in 200
   b. Bowel injury is 2 in 1000
   c. Blood vessel injury is 2 in 1000
   d. Death occurs in 1 in 12,000
   e. Stomach injury 2 in 1000

3. You (specialty trainee year 2) are seeing a 45-year-old woman (Mrs. Smith) in gynaecology clinic. She has menorrhagia. She has regular heavy menstrual bleeding with no intermenstrual or post-coital bleeding. She has had a recent normal cervical smear test result. She has tried a mirena IUS, but it did not work for her. She has also had an endometrial ablation 1 year ago but still has heavy periods. You discuss with your consultant in clinic, who advises to offer her an abdominal hysterectomy. You have never consented for a hysterectomy but have observed your consultant doing it. You go through the RCOG guideline for consent advice for hysterectomy and then go back to see Mrs. Smith in clinic. Mrs. Smith asks you about the risks of hysterectomy while you are waiting for your consultant to arrive as she was busy with another patient.
   Which of the following risks should be most emphasized to the patient?
   a. Burning sensation around the scar
   b. Keloid formation
   c. Numbness and tingling

d. Pain
e. Venous thrombosis

4. You are a specialty trainee year 2. You see a 24-year-old woman (Miss MS) who is referred to the gynaecology clinic with pelvic pain. She complains that the pain starts a few days before her period and it remains until the period lasts every month. She does not have any bowel or bladder symptoms. Her ultrasound scan of pelvis is normal. You discuss with your senior registrar in clinic, who advises that she would need diagnostic laparoscopy to rule out any pelvic pathology such as endometriosis. While you are discussing the risks of diagnostic laparoscopy with Miss Rogers, she asks you the risk of bowel injury that might not be diagnosed at the time of laparoscopy.
   Which of the following options is correct?
   a. 4%
   b. 5%
   c. 6%
   d. 9%
   e. 15%

5. You are a specialty trainee year 2 and are about to consent a woman (Mrs. GS) for elective caesarean section. This is her first pregnancy and she is terrified to have a vaginal delivery as her sister had a bad experience in the past. While you are discussing the risks of surgery, Mrs. GS asks you about risk of emergency hysterectomy during caesarean section. Which of the following options is correct?
   a. 1–2 in 1000 women
   b. 2–3 in 1000 women
   c. 3–4 in 1000 women
   d. 5–6 in 1000 women
   e. 7–8 in 1000 women

6. Which of the following is not a frequent risk associated with elective caesarean section?
   a. Abdominal discomfort following surgery
   b. Haemorrhage
   c. Increased risk of repeat caesarean section when a woman attempts a vaginal delivery in future pregnancies
   d. Intensive care admission
   e. Re-admission to hospital

7. Surgical management of miscarriage should be recommended as first-line management in all except which scenario?
   a. If the background history suggests epilepsy
   b. In the presence of haemodynamic instability
   c. If there is suspicion of gestation trophoblastic disease
   d. In the presence of sepsis
   e. Women presenting with heavy bleeding

8. A 26-year-old woman presents to the early pregnancy unit at 10 weeks gestation with heavy vaginal bleeding. It is her first pregnancy and she is anxious. Her scan 2 weeks earlier revealed a single live intrauterine pregnancy. Speculum and clinical examination reveals an open cervical os with products seen at the os and heavy vaginal bleeding with clots, and her pulse is 110/minute and BP is 90/50 mmHg. You are a specialty trainee year 2 and you discuss with her surgical management of miscarriage in view of heavy bleeding and inevitable miscarriage. She would like to avoid a blood transfusion if possible and would also like to know her risk of having a blood transfusion.

    Which of the following options is correct?
    a.   3 in 1000 cases
    b.   5 in 1000 cases
    c.   10 in 1000 cases
    d.   15 in 1000 cases
    e.   20 in 1000 cases

9. A 28-year-old woman, para 1 (previous caesarean section), attends the early pregnancy unit with a history of 10 weeks amenorrhea and mild vaginal bleeding. Her urinary pregnancy test is positive, and her ultrasound scan reveals a gestation sac of 32 mm with no fetal pole or yolk sac. You are a specialty trainee year 2 and have been asked to review this woman and discuss with her the options for the management of her miscarriage. She opts for surgical management and declines expectant or medical management. She is booked as elective procedure the following day for surgical management of miscarriage. You are undertaking the emergency list under supervision of senior registrar. Following dilatation of cervix, you start using a number 10 suction cannula for suction of products of conception. You see the products of conception in the suction tube but then the bleeding starts to become very heavy with clots.

    Which of the following is not a cause for her bleeding?
    a.   Coagulopathy
    b.   Cervical laceration
    c.   Retained pregnancy tissue
    d.   Uterine contractions
    e.   Uterine perforation

10. A 20-year-old woman, para 0, attends the early pregnancy unit with 8 weeks amenorrhea and mild vaginal bleeding. Her urinary pregnancy test is positive, and her ultrasound scan reveals gestation sac of 32 mm with fetal pole but absent heartbeat. You are specialty trainee year 2 and have been asked to review this woman and discuss with her options for the management of her missed miscarriage. She opts to have surgical management and declines expectant or medical management. She is booked as elective procedure the following day for surgical management of miscarriage. You are doing the emergency list under supervision of senior registrar. While you are discussing risks of the procedure, she asks you the possibility of not removing the products of conception completely.

What is the incidence of retained fetal tissue in her case following surgery?
a. 5 in 1000 women
b. 10 in 1000 women
c. 20 in 1000 women
d. 30 in 1000 women
e. 40 in 1000 women

11. You have been asked to consent a 45-year-old woman who is having a
    total abdominal hysterectomy for a fibroid uterus. She has had no previous
    surgery on her abdomen and no past medical history. Which of the following
    complications is rare?
    a. Bladder injury
    b. Blood transfusion
    c. Bowel injury
    d. Haematoma
    e. Ureteric injury

12. You are assisting your consultant perform a total abdominal hysterectomy,
    and there is concern of a complication with the ureter. What post-operative
    investigation would you request to confirm or refute the complication?
    a. Abdominal ultrasound
    b. Abdominal X-ray
    c. Intravenous urogram
    d. CT abdomen and pelvis
    e. Cystoscopy

13. Regarding electrosurgery, which of the following options is false?
    a. For the safe use of bipolar diathermy, a split return electrode is required
    b. Skin burns are more common with unipolar diathermy
    c. Options to cut, coagulate, desiccate or fulgurate rely on changes in power
        and the electrical waveform
    d. To minimize the effects of muscle and neural stimulation, a return pad is
        used for bipolar diathermy
    e. With unipolar diathermy, the electric current preferentially runs through
        the blood vessels

14. You are assisting your consultant in an operating theatre. You have just
    done an endometrial microwave ablation for menorrhagia, and now you are
    performing a laparoscopic bilateral tubal ligation on the same patient. You
    notice there is a white patch on the bowel in the pouch of Douglas. What is the
    correct next step?
    a. Catheterize the patient for 14 days
    b. Continue with the salpingectomy
    c. Hysteroscopy
    d. Laparotomy
    e. Catheterize the patient for 21 days

15. You are with your consultant in an operating theatre, and you are performing a laparoscopy for chronic pelvic pain. Upon insertion of the camera, you notice a bladder injury. What is the correct management?
    a. Catheterize the patient for 14 days
    b. Continue with the salpingectomy
    c. Hysteroscopy
    d. Laparotomy
    e. Catheterize the patient for 21 days

16. You are about to consent a patient for a diagnostic laparoscopy for chronic pelvic pain. She is 25 years old and has no past medical history and is not on any medication. This is her first procedure, and she is very worried and stressed about it. She wants to know the chances of death due to laparoscopy. Which of the following options is correct?
    a. 1–3 in 100,000 women
    b. 3–8 in 100,000 women
    c. 8–13 in 100,000 women
    d. 13–18 in 100,000 women
    e. 18–23 in 100,000 women

17. You are about to consent a patient for a hysteroscopy for menorrhagia. She is 25 years old and has no past medical history and is not on any medication. This is her first procedure, and she is very worried and stressed about it. She wants to know the chances of death due to hysteroscopy. Which of the following options is correct?
    a. 1–3 in 100,000 women
    b. 3–8 in 100,000 women
    c. 8–13 in 100,000 women
    d. 13–18 in 100,000 women
    e. 18–23 in 100,000 women

18. You are about to consent a patient for a caesarean section for failure to progress at 8 cm. She is 25 years old and has no past medical history and is not on any medication. This is her first procedure, and she is very worried and stressed about it. She wants to know the chances of death due to a caesarean section. Which of the following options is correct?
    a. 1 in 12,000 women
    b. 2 in 12,000 women
    c. 3 in 12,000 women
    d. 4 in 12,000 women
    e. 5 in 12,000 women

ANSWERS

1. b.   1 in 200 procedures

Sterilization	
Sterilization should be performed at an interval following any outcome of pregnancy (abortion, vaginal delivery, caesarean section). There is a possibility that the risk of failure is higher when performed during post-partum period, during caesarean section or immediately following or during an abortion. This is important when counselling patients.	
Failure rate of female sterilization	
Laparoscopic sterilization	• The failure rate of laparoscopic sterilization is 2–5 in 1000 procedures at 10 years (uncommon)
Hysteroscopic sterilization	• The failure rate of hysteroscopic sterilization is around 2 in 1000 (uncommon), although there is limited long-term data
Note: The failure rate with sterilization is higher than the failure rate of implants or intrauterine devices (long-acting reversible contraception)	
Male sterilization	
Vasectomy	Risk of failure after male sterilization (vasectomy) is 1 in 2000

Further reading

● Royal College of Obstetricians and Gynaecologists (RCOG). Consent Advice No. 3. Female sterilization. February 2016.

2. a.   Bladder injury is 1 in 200
   Risks of laparoscopic sterilization
   ● Visceral or vessel injury is 2 in 1000 (uncommon).
   ● Death is rare due to this procedure but can occur in 1 in 12,000 cases (very rare).
   ● Failure to complete the procedure is a risk, but exact risk is not quoted in any study.
   ● The risk of laparotomy is 3 in 1000.

Further reading

● Royal College of Obstetricians and Gynaecologists (RCOG). Consent Advice No. 3. Female sterilization. February 2016.

3. e.   Venous thrombosis
   Venous thrombosis is a serious risk

Information on risk

Term	Equivalent numerical ratio
Very common	1/1 to 1/10
Common	1/10 to 1/100
Uncommon	1/100 to 1/1000
Rare	1/1000 to 1/10,000
Very rare	Less than 1/10,000

The risks at hysterectomy are broadly classified as frequent and serious risks

Frequent risks	Serious risks
Pain	Damage to bladder or ureter (7 in 1000)
Bruising	Damage to bowel (4 in 10,000)
Wound infection and delayed wound healing	Haemorrhage needing transfusion (23 in 1000)
Numbness and tingling	Return to theatre (7 in 1000)
Keloid formation	Pelvic abscess/infection (2 in 1000)
Burning sensation around the scar	Venous thromboembolism and PE (4 in 1000)
Urinary tract infection and frequency of micturition	Risk of death within 6 weeks (32 in 100,000)
Ovarian failure	

- One should always discuss not only procedure (abdominal hysterectomy) but also additional procedures, which may be required during this procedure (blood transfusion, repair of injured organs and oophorectomy for unexpected cause).

Further reading

- Royal College of Obstetricians and Gynaecologists (RCOG). Consent Advice No. 4. Abdominal hysterectomy for benign conditions. May 2009.

4. e.   15%

Diagnostic laparoscopy	
Serious complications	• Serious complications from diagnostic laparoscopy are around 2 per 1000 women (injury to bowel, bladder, ureter, vessels and uterus) • The risk of bowel injury which may not be diagnosed at the time of laparoscopy is around 15%
Frequent risks	• Frequent risks include bruising, shoulder tip pain, infection and wound gape
Additional procedures	• Additional procedures that need consent include blood transfusion, laparotomy and repair of injured organs (bowel, bladder, ureter, vessels)

Further reading

- Royal College of Obstetricians and Gynaecologists (RCOG). Consent Advice No. 2. Diagnostic laparoscopy. June 2017.

5. e.   7–8 in 1000 women

Serious risks of having a caesarean section include the following

Need for further surgery, including curettage	5 in 1000 women
Admission to intensive care unit	9 in 1000 women
Thromboembolism	4–16 in 10,000 women (rare)
Bladder injury	1 in 1000 women
Ureteric injury	3 in 10,000 women (rare)
Death	1 in 12,000 women (very rare)
Emergency hysterectomy	7–8 in 1000 women

Further reading

- Royal College of Obstetricians and Gynaecologists (RCOG). Consent Advice No. 7. Caesarean section. October 2009.

6. d.   Intensive care admission

Frequent risks associated with caesarean section (CS) include the following:

Maternal frequent risks	
Persistent wound or abdominal discomfort in first few months following CS	9 in 100 women
Increased risk of CS in next pregnancy when women attempt to have vaginal delivery	1 in 4 women
Re-admission to hospital	5 in 100 women
Haemorrhage	5 in 1000 women
Infection	6 in 100 women
Fetal frequent risks	
Laceration	1–2 in 100 women

Further reading

- Royal College of Obstetricians and Gynaecologists (RCOG). Consent Advice No. 7. Caesarean section. October 2009.

7. a.   If the background history suggests epilepsy

Expectant management for the first 7–14 days is recommended by National Institute of Clinical Excellence (NICE) in women with established diagnosis of miscarriage. Medical or expectant management should be offered when expectant management has failed or is not acceptable to the women. Surgical management should be first-line management in women with sepsis, suspicion of molar pregnancy or women presenting with heavy bleeding and/or being haemodynamically unstable with tachycardia or hypotension.

Further reading

- Royal College of Obstetricians and Gynaecologists (RCOG). Consent Advice No. 10. Surgical Management of Miscarriage and Removal of Persistent Placental or Fetal Remains (Consent Advice No. 10—Joint with AEPU). January 2018.

8. a. 3 in 1000 cases

Women requiring blood transfusion due to heavy bleeding is not common and quoted incidence is 0–3 in 1000 cases.

Further reading

- Royal College of Obstetricians and Gynaecologists (RCOG). Consent Advice No. 10. Surgical Management of Miscarriage and Removal of Persistent Placental or Fetal Remains (Consent Advice No. 10—Joint with AEPU). January 2018.

9. d. Uterine contractions

Surgical management of miscarriage (heavy bleeding during or after surgery)

Reasons for heavy bleeding during or shortly after surgical management of miscarriage	• Bleeding during or shortly following procedure can be caused by atony of uterus, coagulopathy or abnormal placentation • Complication such as uterine perforation, cervical laceration and retained pregnancy tissue need to be thought in her case as these are common causes of heavy bleeding. All three reasons can occur in her case • Although bleeding is unexpected in women with history of previous caesarean section, a possibility of undiagnosed caesarean scar pregnancy need to be ruled out • Also, one needs to think of some early cases of gestational trophoblastic disease that are not detected by ultrasound scan when there is unexpected bleeding
Bleeding lasting for more than 2 weeks	• Incomplete evacuation or incomplete procedure or retained placental or fetal tissue needs to be ruled out if the bleeding persists for >2 weeks post-surgery

a. The risk of cervical trauma may be reduced by cervical priming with prostaglandins. One needs to consider this especially in nulliparous women who have had no bleeding or only mild bleeding prior to the procedure. The incidence of cervical trauma is 1 in 1000 women (uncommon).

b. The incidence of confirmed perforation is 1 in 1000 women. As many perforations may not be diagnosed at the time of surgery, the incidence can be as high as 15 in 1000 women as per observational study.

c. Most perforations are usually small, and conservative management is enough to manage such cases. If surrounding organ damage (bowel, bladder damage) is suspected or there is heavy bleeding, then a laparoscopy and or laparotomy would be necessary to repair the damage and manage the complication.

Further reading

- Royal College of Obstetricians and Gynaecologists (RCOG). Consent Advice No. 10. Surgical Management of Miscarriage and Removal of Persistent Placental or Fetal Remains (Consent Advice No. 10—Joint with AEPU). January 2018.

10. e. 40 in 1000 women

Women should be adequately counselled regarding risks of surgical management of miscarriage, including the possibility of an incomplete procedure or retained products of conception (40 in 1000 women) and need for further repeat surgery following surgical evacuation of the uterus (3 in 1000 women).

Randomized controlled trials have shown that the incidence of incomplete procedure or retained products of conception can be reduced with appropriate use of transvaginal ultrasound in theatre once the surgery is accomplished. However, the limitations include the need for a high-resolution ultrasound scan machine and the expertise to use the scan machine.

Further reading

- Royal College of Obstetricians and Gynaecologists (RCOG). Consent Advice No. 10. Surgical Management of Miscarriage and Removal of Persistent Placental or Fetal Remains (Consent Advice No. 10—Joint with AEPU). January 2018.

11. c. Bowel injury

The risks of bladder injury, pulmonary embolus and pelvic abscess are uncommon (1/100–1/1000), whereas bowel injury is rare (1/1000–1/10,000). The risk of blood transfusion is common (1/10–1/100).

Further reading

- Royal College of Obstetricians and Gynaecologists. *Abdominal Hysterectomy for Benign Conditions: Consent Advice No. 4.* London, UK: RCOG, 2009.
- Raghavan R, Arya P, Arya P, China S. Abdominal incisions and sutures in obstetrics and gynaecology. *The Obstetrician & Gynaecologist* 2014; 16:13–18.

12. c. Intravenous urogram

The ideal investigation is an intravenous urogram. CT and ultrasound will not pick up a small injury, and the cystoscopy will not investigate the appropriate organ.

Further reading

* RCOG online learning resource: StratOG: Abdominal Surgery.
* Brown SR, Goodfellow PB. Transverse verses midline incisions for abdominal surgery. *Cochrane Database Systematische Reviews* 2005; 4:CD005199.

13. a.   For the safe use of bipolar diathermy, a split return electrode is required
    In bipolar diathermy, the current flows between the electrodes and does not run through the body. Therefore, a return electrode is not required.
    With unipolar diathermy, the current runs from the electrode, preferentially through the vascular tree towards the return electrode (usually located over the quadriceps muscle). If there is poor contact, burns will occur on the skin at the site of the return electrode. Burns are therefore more common.
    To minimize the effects of muscle and neural stimulation, electrosurgical equipment typically operates at a frequency of 100 kHz to 5 MHz.

Further reading

* RCOG online learning resource: StratOG: Abdominal Surgery.
* World Health Organization. *Implementation Manual/WHO Surgical Safety Checklist 2009* [Accessed August 2019].

14. d.   Laparotomy
    There is a thermal injury to the bowel; therefore, the correct treatment is laparotomy and repair.

Further reading

* RCOG online learning resource: StratOG: Abdominal Surgery.
* Royal College of Obstetricians and Gynaecologists. *Preventing Entry-Related Gynaecological Laparoscopic Injuries: Green-top Guideline 49.* London, UK: RCOG, 2008.

15. a.   Catheterize the patient for 14 days
    The bladder needs time to heal and therefore 2 weeks with the catheter should be sufficient.

Further reading

* RCOG online learning resource: StratOG: Abdominal Surgery.
* Kalu G, Wright J. Laparoscopic surgery and the law. *The Obstetrician & Gynaecologist* 2001; 3:141–146.

16. b.   3–8 in 100,000 women
    Death is very rare, affecting 3–8 in 100,000 women undergoing a laparoscopy.

Further reading

* Royal College of Obstetricians and Gynaecologists. *Diagnostic Laparoscopy: Consent Advice No. 2.* London, UK: RCOG, 2017.

- Ewen SP. Avoiding complications of the laparoscopic approach. *The Obstetrician & Gynaecologist* 1999; 1:34–36.

17. b.   3–8 in 100,000 women
3–8 in 10,000 women will die when undergoing a hysteroscopy.

Further reading

- Royal College of Obstetricians and Gynaecologists. *Diagnostic Hysteroscopy Under General Anaesthesia: Consent Advice No. 1.* London, UK: RCOG, 2008.
- Cooper NAM, Clark TJ. Ambulatory hysteroscopy. *The Obstetrician & Gynaecologist* 2013; 15:159–166.

18. a.   1 in 12,000 women
The risk of death with a caesarean section is approximately 1 in every 12,000 women (very rare).

Further reading

- Royal College of Obstetricians and Gynaecologists. Cesarean section. Consent Advise No. 7. 2009.
- National Institute for Health and Clinical Excellence. *Caesarean Section: Clinical Guideline 132.* London, UK: NICE, 2011.

QUESTIONS

1. What is the 30-day mortality risk for high-risk patients who received inadequate pre-operative fluid management, compared to those with adequate pre-operative fluid management?
   a. 10%
   b. 20%
   c. 30%
   d. 40%
   e. 50%

2. Before any operation, antibiotics should be given. How many minutes prior to the surgery is the optimal time for the antibiotics to be given?
   a. 0–15 minutes
   b. 15–60 minutes
   c. 60–75 minutes
   d. 75–90 minutes
   e. 90–180 minutes

3. You are the senior house officer (SHO) on labour ward, and you have been asked to see a patient who just came out of theatre following an emergency caesarean section for failure to progress at 5 cm dilation. She is otherwise obstetrically low risk. You review her and note that she is haemodynamically stable and that it was an uncomplicated section with only 200 mL blood loss. The nurse in charge is asking when the patient can start taking in oral fluids. What is your answer?
   a. Immediately
   b. In 30 minutes
   c. In 60 minutes
   d. In 90 minutes
   e. Only when the catheter has been removed and she has passed urine

4. You have been asked to review a 42-year-old woman who had a total abdominal hysterectomy for a fibroid uterus 12 hours ago. She has a temperature of 38°C. All other observations were normal. What is the most likely diagnosis?
   a. Deep vein
   b. Haematoma

    c. Pulmonary atelectasis
    d. Pulmonary embolism
    e. Urinary tract infection

5. In which of the following procedures is antibiotic prophylaxis not recommended?
    a. Caesarean section
    b. Instrumental delivery
    c. Subtotal abdominal hysterectomy
    d. Total abdominal hysterectomy
    e. Vaginal hysterectomy

6. What is the most important factor of enhanced recovery?
    a. Carbohydrate meal prior to surgery
    b. Early mobilization
    c. Intraoperative fluids
    d. Post-operative fluids
    e. To eat immediately after surgery

7. You are covering the postnatal ward and the midwife is asking you if a patient needs postnatal thromboprophylaxis. She is 25 years old and is now a para 1 after having an emergency caesarean for failure to progress at 8 cm. Her BMI is 25, she has no past medical history and she is not on any medication. What is the correct answer?
    a. 10 days of prophylactic low–molecular-weight heparin
    b. 14 days of prophylactic low–molecular-weight heparin
    c. 6 weeks of prophylactic low–molecular-weight heparin
    d. Discuss with a haematologist
    e. No need of prophylactic low–molecular-weight heparin

8. You are covering the postnatal ward, and the midwife is asking you if a patient needs postnatal thromboprophylaxis. She is 36 years old and is now a para 3 after having a forceps delivery. She has a BMI of 25, has no past medical history and is not on any medication. What is the correct answer? What is your management plan for this woman regarding thromboprophylaxis?
    a. 10 days of prophylactic low–molecular-weight heparin
    b. 14 days of prophylactic low–molecular-weight heparin
    c. 6 weeks of prophylactic low–molecular-weight heparin
    d. Discuss with a haematologist
    e. No need of prophylactic low–molecular-weight heparin

ANSWERS

1. b. 20%
It is approximately five times higher.

Further reading

- RCOG online learning resource. StratOG: Routine post-operative care.
- National Institute for Health and Care Excellence. *Intravenous Fluid Therapy in Adults in Hospital: CG174.* NICE, 2013 (updated 2017).

2. b. 15–60 minutes

Further reading

- RCOG online learning resource. StratOG: Routine post-operative care.
- National Institute for Health and Care Excellence. *Surgical Site Infection: Prevention and Treatment of Surgical Site Infection.* CG74. London, UK: NICE, 2017.

3. a. Immediately
Oral fluids can be started immediately as it will help in recovery, provided she is not vomiting.

Further reading

- RCOG online learning resource. StratOG: Routine post-operative care.
- Torbe E, Crawford R, Norbin A, Acheson N. Enhanced recovery in gynaecology. *The Obstetrician & Gynaecologist* 2013; 15:263–268.

4. c. Pulmonary atelectasis
At 12 hours post GA, the most likely diagnosis is pulmonary atelectasis.

Further reading

- RCOG online learning resource. StratOG: Routine post-operative care.
- Royal College of Obstetricians and Gynaecologists. *Enhanced Recovery in Gynaecology. Scientific Impact Paper No. 36.* London, UK: RCOG, 2013.

5. b. Instrumental delivery
When preforming an instrumental delivery, antibiotics are not required. All other procedures require antibiotics.

Further reading

- Scottish Intercollegiate Guidelines Network. *Antibiotic Prophylaxis in Surgery. SIGN Guideline 104.* Edinburgh, Scotland: SIGN, 2014.
- National Institute for Health and Clinical Excellence. *Routine Preoperative Tests for Elective Surgery. NG45.* London, UK: NICE, 2016.

6. b. Early mobilization
Early mobilization prevents impaired lung function, reduces the risk of thromboembolism and increased insulin resistance. Therefore, the most important factor in enhanced recovery is early mobilization.

Further reading

- National Confidential Enquiry into Patient Outcome and Death. Knowing the risk. *A Review of the Peri-operative Care of Surgical Patients*. London, UK: NCEPOD, 2011.
- NHS Improvement. *Enhanced Recovery—Gynaecology*. www.nhs.uk.

7. a. 10 days of prophylactic low–molecular-weight heparin
Ten days prophylaxis with low–molecular-weight heparin is recommended for low-risk women who have an emergency caesarean section in labour.

Further reading

- RCOG Green Top guideline. 37a. *Reducing the Risk of Venous Thromboembolism During Pregnancy and the Puerperium*. London, UK: RCOG, April 2015.

8. a. 10 days of prophylactic low–molecular-weight heparin
This patient has two risk factors (instrumental delivery and para 3) and therefore qualifies for 10 days of prophylactic low–molecular-weight heparin.

Further reading

- RCOG Green Top guideline. 37a. *Reducing the Risk of Venous Thromboembolism during Pregnancy and the Puerperium*. London, UK: RCOG, April 2015.

KNOWLEDGE AREA 5: ANTENATAL CARE

QUESTIONS

1. Trisomy 18 has which of the following features?
   a. Congenital stomach defects
   b. Flexion of hands and fingers
   c. High-set deformed ears
   d. "Lemon-shaped" head
   e. Macrognathia

2. A 23-year-old woman just delivered a baby boy. It was noted that he has large ears, large testes and a prominent jaw. The paediatrician tells the parents that it is likely this child will have learning difficulties. Which of the following is the most likely diagnosis?
   a. Down syndrome
   b. Edwards syndrome
   c. Fragile X syndrome
   d. Pfeiffer syndrome
   e. Turner syndrome

3. Which of the following is correctly matched with regard to development of external genitalia in females?
   a. Genital tubercle – mons pubis
   b. Genital folds – labia minora
   c. Genital swellings – mons pubis
   d. Genital swellings – clitoris
   e. Urogenital grove – clitoris

4. Which of the following best describes the paramesonephric duct?
   a. Caudally, opens into the abdominal cavity
   b. Caudally, it runs superior to the mesonephric duct before it crosses it
   c. Caudally, it runs medial to the mesonephric duct, after crossing it ventrally
   d. Caudally, it runs laterally to the mesonephric duct, after crossing it
   e. In midline, it fuses with the opposite mesonephric duct

5. Which of the following is true about blood pressure changes during pregnancy?
   a. Blood pressure is lower in the supine position than sitting position
   b. Blood pressure is higher in the supine position than sitting position

   c.   Diastolic pressure is increased in mid-trimester

   d.   Systolic pressure changes throughout pregnancy

   e.   There is an increase in peripheral vascular resistance

6. A 33-year-old pregnant woman with hypothyroidism comes to see you in the antenatal clinic during the second trimester of pregnancy. Which of the following is true regarding the changes in serum thyroid hormone levels in pregnancy?

   a.   Free T4 is decreased during second trimester

   b.   Serum thyroglobulin level is increased

   c.   Total T3 level is decreased

   d.   Total T4 level is unchanged

   e.   Total T4 level is decreased

7. Which of the following is true regarding the physiological changes of blood and blood flow during pregnancy?

   a.   Blood flow to the kidneys is increased to 700 mL/min

   b.   Blood flow to the uterus is increased to 700 mL/min

   c.   Plasma volume is increased by 70%

   d.   Plasma volume reaches a plateau around 20 weeks

   e.   Red cell volume is increased by 60%

8. If taken antenatally, which of the following drugs causes nasal hypoplasia, recurrent intracranial haemorrhage and chondrodysplasia punctate?

   a.   Aspirin

   b.   Atenolol

   c.   Bromocriptine

   d.   Sodium valproate

   e.   Warfarin

9. You have been asked to investigate the perinatal death rate in your unit. How is this defined?

   a.   Stillbirths plus first week deaths per 1000 live births

   b.   Stillbirths plus first week deaths per 1000 live births and stillbirths

   c.   Stillbirths plus first 2 weeks deaths per 1000 live births

   d.   Stillbirths plus first 2 weeks deaths per 1000 live births and stillbirths

   e.   None of the above

10. Which of the following regarding neonatal deaths is true?

   a.   Early neonatal death is death at 0–30 days of life

   b.   Early neonatal death is death at 0–8 days of life

   c.   Late neonatal deaths are deaths after 30 days of life

   d.   Neonatal death rate is the number of deaths at 0–27 days per 1000 live births

   e.   Post-neonatal deaths are deaths at >28 days of life but <6 months

11. Regarding maternal death, which of the following is true?
    a. Coincidental deaths are those that occur during pregnancy due to causes not related to pregnancy
    b. Direct deaths are those resulting from previously existing disease leading to death during pregnancy
    c. Indirect deaths are deaths resulting from conditions that are unique to pregnancy and these may occur during antepartum, intrapartum and postpartum periods
    d. Is death of women while pregnant or within 30 days of termination of pregnancy or from any cause related to or aggravated by the pregnancy or its management
    e. Late deaths are those that occur between 42 days and 6 months of termination of pregnancy, miscarriage or delivery, which are due to direct or indirect maternal causes

12. Which of the following is *not* due to non-dysjunction during meiosis?
    a. Down syndrome
    b. Edwards syndrome
    c. Klinefelter syndrome
    d. Prader–Willi syndrome
    e. Turner syndrome

13. A 28-year-old primigravida comes to see you in the antenatal clinic at 32 weeks of pregnancy. She is worried because she has just found out that her cousin is a carrier of the cystic fibrosis gene. What is its inheritance pattern?
    a. Autosomal dominant
    b. Autosomal recessive
    c. Mitochondrial
    d. X-linked dominant
    e. X-linked recessive

14. Which of the following is X-linked recessive condition?
    a. Familial hypercholesterolemia
    b. Glucose-6-phosphate dehydrogenase
    c. Huntington's disease
    d. Sickle cell disease
    e. Vitamin D-resistant rickets

15. A 22-year-old woman with achondroplasia comes to see you in the antenatal clinic. Her partner does not have achondroplasia. She would like to know the chances of her child inheriting this condition?
    a. 0%
    b. 25%
    c. 50%
    d. 75%
    e. 100%

ANSWERS

1. b.   Flexion of hands and fingers

Trisomy 18 is also called Edwards syndrome. The incidence is 1:5000 newborns. Fetal loss (85%) usually occurs between 10 weeks of gestation and term, and those born alive usually die within 2 months (10% survive to 1 year). In addition to the features described, it is associated with abnormalities of the skeletal system, omphalocele, intrauterine growth retardation and severe learning disability.

Further reading

- Sarris I, Sangeeta A, Susan B. *Training in Obstetrics and Gynaecology: The Essential Curriculum.* Oxford, UK: Oxford University Press, 2009, pp. 391–416.

2. c.   Fragile X syndrome

Fragile X syndrome

- Fragile X syndrome is more common in males than females
- The incidence in males is 1:1000, while in females it is 1:2000
- While considering the cause for learning disability due to chromosomal abnormalities, fragile X syndrome stands second to Down syndrome
- It is characterized by learning disability, large ears, large testes and a prominent jaw
- The fragile site on the long arm of the X chromosome (Xq27) has been correlated with the altered phenotype and is called fragile X syndrome
- The regions on the chromosome that are vulnerable to separate or break under certain manipulations are called the fragile site

---

Further reading

- Sarris I, Sangeeta A, Susan B. *Training in Obstetrics and Gynaecology: The Essential Curriculum.* Oxford, UK: Oxford University Press, 2009, pp. 391–416.

3. b.   Genital folds – labia minora

The mons pubis arises from genital swellings. In females, the genital fold gives rise to the labia minora, and in males, the genital fold gives rise to ventral aspect of the penis. In females, the genital swellings give rise to the labia majora, and in males, the genital swellings give rise to scrotum. The urogenital grove gives rise to the vestibule. The clitoris arises from the genital tubercle.

Further reading

- Sarris I, Sangeeta A, Susan B. *Training in Obstetrics and Gynaecology: The Essential Curriculum.* Oxford, UK: Oxford University Press, 2009, pp. 391–416.

4. c. Caudally, it runs medial to the mesonephric duct, after crossing it ventrally

There are two mesonephric ducts (Wolffian duct system) and two paramesonephric ducts (Mullerian duct system) in the body during embryonic development of the reproductive organs. The paramesonephric duct arises from the invagination of the epithelium covering the urogenital ridge on the anterolateral surface. It opens cranially into the abdominal cavity. Caudally, it lies lateral to the mesonephric duct before crossing it ventrally. It then lies medial to the mesonephric duct. Further to this, it joins the opposite paramesonephric duct in the midline and forms the uterine cavity. In females, the paramesonephric duct gives rise to the uterus, fallopian tubes, cervix, upper third of the vagina (lower two-thirds of the vagina develop from urogenital sinus) and a vestigial or rudimentary structure called Morgagni hydatid. In males, it forms the vestigial structure called the appendix of testis.

Further reading

● Sarris I, Sangeeta A, Susan B. *Training in Obstetrics and Gynaecology: The Essential Curriculum.* Oxford, UK: Oxford University Press, 2009, pp. 391–416.

5. a. Blood pressure is lower in the supine position than sitting position

Diastolic pressure is reduced in mid-trimester. Systolic blood pressure is unchanged during pregnancy. There is decrease in peripheral vascular resistance. The blood pressure is lower in the supine than in the sitting position.

Further reading

● Sarris I, Sangeeta A, Susan B. *Training in Obstetrics and Gynaecology: The Essential Curriculum.* Oxford, UK: Oxford University Press, 2009, pp. 391–416.

6. b. Serum thyroglobulin level is increased

Both total T4 level and total T3 level are increased. Free T4 is unchanged during second trimester. There is an increase in vascularity and the size of the thyroid gland. Thyroid-binding globulin also increases during pregnancy.

Due to increase in GFR, the loss of iodine in the urine is increased. This loss is not reflected in the serum iodine levels unless the pregnant woman is iodine deficient (there is no reduction in the serum iodine).

Further reading

● Sarris I, Sangeeta A, Susan B. *Training in Obstetrics and Gynaecology: The Essential Curriculum.* Oxford, UK: Oxford University Press, 2009, pp. 391–416.

7. b. Blood flow to the uterus is increased to 700 mL/min

During pregnancy, plasma volume is increased by 50% and the red cell volume increases by 40%. Plasma volume reaches a plateau around 32–34 weeks.

The blood flow to various organs is increased, for example, uterus (700 mL/min), skin (500 mL/min) and kidneys (400 mL/min). There is a threefold increase in erythropoietin levels, and this is associated with an increase in red blood cell mass (40% rise) and also with an increase in fetal haemoglobin. Since the plasma volume expansion is more than the red blood cell mass, there is a fall in the haemoglobin and haematocrit levels. There is also decrease in the plasma proteins in the circulation, which leads to fall in plasma oncotic pressure but there is rise in circulating venous pressure. This contributes to the oedema during pregnancy.

Further reading

- Sarris I, Sangeeta A, Susan B. *Training in Obstetrics and Gynaecology: The Essential Curriculum.* Oxford, UK: Oxford University Press, 2009, pp. 391–416.
- Soma-Pillay P, Catherine NP, Tolppanen H, Mebazaa A, Tolppanen H, Mebazaa A. Physiological changes in pregnancy. *Cardiovasc Journal of Africa* 2016; 27(2):89–94.

8. e. Warfarin

Warfarin is teratogenic to the fetus. It is an anticoagulant and should be stopped during pregnancy due to its effects on the fetus. It can be replaced with clexane during pregnancy. Warfarin can cause the following fetal abnormalities:

- CNS abnormalities (due to recurrent bleeds)
- Nasal hypoplasia
- Chondrodysplasia punctata (stippled bone epiphysis)
- Intrauterine growth retardation
- Neurodevelopmental delay
- Learning disability
- Malformations of the vertebral body

These are collectively called warfarin embryopathy.

Further reading

- Sarris I, Sangeeta A, Susan B. *Training in Obstetrics and Gynaecology: The Essential Curriculum.* Oxford, UK: Oxford University Press, 2009, pp. 391–416.
- https://en.wikipedia.org/wiki/Fetal_warfarin_syndrome

9. b. Stillbirths plus first week deaths per 1000 live births and stillbirths

Perinatal death rate is the number of stillbirths plus first week deaths per 1000 live births and stillbirths.

Reference

- Lewis, G (ed). The confidential enquiry into maternal and child health (CEMACH). Saving Mothers' Lives: Reviewing maternal deaths to make motherhood safer—2003–2005. *The Seventh Report on Confidential Enquiries into Maternal Deaths in the United Kingdom.* London, UK: CEMACH, 2007. Available at: www.cmace.org.uk.

10. d.   Neonatal death rate is the number of deaths at 0–27 days per 1000 live births
Definitions

Early neonatal deaths	Are deaths that occur between 0 and 6 days of life
Early neonatal death rate	Is the number of deaths at 0–6 days per 1000 live births
Late neonatal deaths	Are deaths occurring between 7 and 27 days of life
Late neonatal death rate	Is the number of deaths at 7–27 days per 1000 live births
Neonatal deaths	Are deaths occurring between 0 and 27 days of life
Neonatal death rate	Is the number of deaths occurring between 0 and 27 days per 1000 live births
Post-neonatal deaths	Are deaths after 28 days of life and <1 year of life
Post-neonatal death rate	Is the number of deaths >28 days but <1 year per 1000 live births

Further reading

- Lewis, G (ed). The confidential enquiry into maternal and child health (CEMACH). Saving Mothers' Lives: Reviewing maternal deaths to make motherhood safer—2003–2005. *The Seventh Report on Confidential Enquiries into Maternal Deaths in the United Kingdom.* London, UK: CEMACH, 2007.
- www.cmace.org.uk.

11. a.   Coincidental deaths are those that occur during pregnancy due to causes not related to pregnancy

Definitions and classification of maternal deaths	
Maternal death is death of women while pregnant or within 42 days of termination of pregnancy or from any cause related to or aggravated by the pregnancy or its management	
Direct	Are deaths resulting from obstetric complications of the pregnant state (pregnancy, labour and puerperium), from interventions, omissions, incorrect treatment, or from a chain of events resulting from any of the above
Indirect	Are deaths resulting from previous existing disease, or disease that developed during pregnancy and that was not due to direct obstetric causes, but was aggravated by the physiological effects of pregnancy
Late	Are deaths occurring between 42 days and 1 year after abortion, miscarriage or deliveries that are due to direct or indirect maternal causes
Coincidental or fortuitous	Are deaths from unrelated causes that happen to occur in pregnancy or the puerperium

Further reading

- Lewis, G (ed). The confidential enquiry into maternal and child health (CEMACH). Saving Mothers' Lives: Reviewing maternal deaths to make motherhood safer—2003–2005. *The Seventh Report on Confidential Enquiries into Maternal Deaths in the United Kingdom.* London, UK: CEMACH, 2007.
- Available at: www.cmace.org.uk.

12. d.   Prader–Willi syndrome

Medical syndromes and genetic reasons for these syndromes	
Prader–Willi syndrome	• First described by Swiss doctors A. Prader, A. Labhart and H. Willi • Is a rare genetic disease • The majority are caused by deletion on chromosome 15, which is inherited from the father, and the rest are caused by inheriting two chromosome 15 from the mother • Is characterized by obesity • Excessive eating (hyperphagia) • Short stature, small hands and feet • Hypotonia and hypogonadism
Down syndrome (trisomy 21)	Is due to non-dysjunction during meiosis
Edwards (trisomy 18)	Is due to non-dysjunction during meiosis
Turner syndrome (45 X/45 XO)	Usually due to sporadic chromosomal non-dysjunction
Klinefelter's syndrome (47 XXY)	Is caused by meiotic non-dysjunction of sex chromosome during gametogenesis

Further reading

● Sarris I, Sangeeta A, Susan B. *Training in Obstetrics and Gynaecology: The Essential Curriculum.* Oxford, UK: Oxford University Press, 2009, pp. 391–416.

13. b.   Autosomal recessive

The mode of inheritance of cystic fibrosis is autosomal recessive. The defect is on the chromosome 7 CFTR gene. There is lack of Cl⁻ transport and failure to hydrate the mucous secretions, which leads to thick viscous mucoid secretions.

The following are the complications of cystic fibrosis in fetus and later in life:

● Meconium ileus caused by thick meconium
● Respiratory distress due to bronchiectasis
● Pancreatic insufficiency
● Pseudomonas pneumonia

Autosomal recessive disorders

• Acute fatty liver of pregnancy	• Donohue syndrome	• Gastroschisis
• Acyl-CoA oxidase deficiency	• DOOR syndrome	• Gaucher's disease
• Adenine phosphoribosyltransferase deficiency	• Dopamine beta-hydroxylase deficiency	• Glutathione synthetase deficiency
• Adenosine deaminase 2 deficiency	• Dubin–Johnson syndrome	• Glycine encephalopathy
• Adenylosuccinate lyase deficiency	• Dubowitz syndrome	• Glycogen storage disease type I–III
• Albinism in humans	• Essential fructosuria	• Glycogen storage disease type V
• Aldolase A deficiency	• Familial Mediterranean fever	• Phosphofructokinase deficiency
• Alkaptonuria	• Fanconi anaemia	• GM1 gangliosidoses
• Bloom syndrome	• Follicle-stimulating hormone insensitivity	• GM2 gangliosidoses
• Chédiak–Higashi syndrome	• Fraser syndrome	• GM2 gangliosidosis, AB variant
• Congenital adrenal hyperplasia due to 21-hydroxylase deficiency	• Friedreich's ataxia	• Gonadotropin-releasing hormone insensitivity
• Cystathioninuria	• Fumarase deficiency	• Gunther disease
• Cystinuria	• Galactokinase deficiency	• Histidinaemia
	• Galactose-1-phosphate uridylyltransferase deficiency	• Homocystinuria
	• Galactosialidosis	• Hurler syndrome
	• Gangliosidosis	• Mucopolysaccharidosis type I

Further reading

- Sarris I, Sangeeta A, Susan B. *Training in Obstetrics and Gynaecology: The Essential Curriculum.* Oxford, UK: Oxford University Press, 2009, pp. 391–416.
- https://en.wikipedia.org/wiki/Category:Autosomal_recessive_disorders

14. b. Glucose-6-phosphate dehydrogenase
    - Familial hypercholesterolemia and Huntington's disease – autosomal dominant.
    - Sickle cell disease – autosomal recessive
    - Vitamin D-resistant rickets – X-linked dominant
    - Familial hypercholesterolaemia – autosomal dominant

Further reading

- Sarris I, Sangeeta A, Susan B. *Training in Obstetrics and Gynaecology: The Essential Curriculum.* Oxford, UK: Oxford University Press, 2009, pp. 391–416.
- https://en.wikipedia.org/wiki/Glucose-6-phosphate_dehydrogenase

15. c. 50%

    The condition is inherited in an autosomal dominant fashion; therefore, her child has a 50% chance of inheriting the disorder. Other autosomal dominant conditions are Huntington's disease, neurofibromatosis and familial hypercholesterolaemia.

Further reading

- Sarris I, Sangeeta A, Susan B. *Training in Obstetrics and Gynaecology: The Essential Curriculum.* Oxford, UK: Oxford University Press, 2009, pp. 391–416.
- https://en.wikipedia.org/wiki/Achondroplasia

QUESTIONS

1. A 27-year-old woman in her first pregnancy comes to see you in the antenatal clinic at 23 weeks of gestation. She is worried because she has found a hard, immobile lump whilst examining her right breast. She is very anxious because her mother died of breast cancer.

   How would you manage her?
   a. Chest X-ray and liver ultrasound
   b. Mammography
   c. Tumour markers such as CA15-3, CEA and CA125
   d. Ultrasound-guided biopsy for cytology
   e. Ultrasound-guided biopsy for histology

2. You receive a phone call from the general practitioner (GP). He is asking how long the patient consulting him should wait before getting pregnant. She had bariatric surgery 12 months ago and wants to get pregnant. What would be your answer to him?
   a. Advise against pregnancy altogether
   b. Can attempt to get pregnant anytime from now
   c. Wait another 6 months
   d. Wait another 12 months
   e. Wait another 24 months

3. You are seeing a 37-year-old woman in the antenatal clinic. She has essential hypertension which is well controlled and has been taking chlorothiazide for 7 years. She is currently 8 weeks pregnant and otherwise well.

   Which of the following is the most appropriate recommendations for her?
   a. Change antihypertensive, start 75 mg aspirin, aim to keep BP less than <150/100
   b. Change antihypertensive, start 150 mg aspirin, aim to keep BP less than <150/100
   c. Change antihypertensive, start 75 mg aspirin, aim to keep BP less than <140/90
   d. Do not change antihypertensive, start 75 mg aspirin, aim to keep BP less than <150/100
   e. Do not change antihypertensive, start 150 mg aspirin, aim to keep BP less than <140/90

4. A 32-year-old woman who is currently 27 weeks pregnant attended maternity triage because she hugged her nephew who has chicken pox for the last 5 days. Her serological test shows that the patient is not immune to chicken pox.

   What is the correct management?
   a. Admit patient for steroids
   b. Reassure patient
   c. Repeat serological tests in 1 week
   d. Offer acyclovir
   e. Offer varicella zoster immunoglobulin (VZIG) as soon as possible

5. You are the senior house officer (SHO) on the postnatal ward. You are informed of a patient known to have well-controlled epilepsy who has just delivered. She had an uncomplicated normal vaginal delivery. She is on carbamazepine and is asking your advice for the best contraception for her in the future.

   What would be your recommendation?
   a. Combined hormonal contraception
   b. Levonorgestrel-releasing intrauterine system (LNG-IUS)
   c. Progestogen-only implants
   d. Progestogen-only pills
   e. Transdermal contraceptive patch

6. You are the SHO working in maternity day assessment unit and you have been asked to review a pregnant woman who is at 24 weeks of gestation in her first pregnancy. She is currently complaining of multiple painful lesions on her vulva. You think the diagnosis is genital herpes on examination. She informs you that this is the first time they have appeared.

   What is the correct management plan?
   a. Prescribe acyclovir
   b. Prescribe steroid cream
   c. Reassure patient
   d. Refer to genitourinary medicine (GUM) physician
   e. Take blood testing for full blood count, urea and electrolytes and C-reactive protein

7. You are in the antenatal clinic and you review a 23-year-old woman who is 8 weeks pregnant. She is known to have Eisenmenger's syndrome. She has been told that there is a significant mortality associated with this condition in pregnancy and she would like to discuss that risk.

   What is mortality risk for her?
   a. 0%–20%
   b. 20%–40%
   c. 40%–60%
   d. 60%–80%
   e. 80%–100%

8. You are the SHO in maternity triage or obstetric day assessment unit. A 36-week pregnant patient presents with sudden onset of epigastric pain

which radiates through to her back. She has vomited four times over the last 6 hours and feels very nauseous. The midwives sent some blood tests which revealed a raised amylase (1000 units/L) with normal liver function tests.

What is your initial management?

a. Urinary catheter, analgesia and consider induction of labour
b. Intravenous fluid and oxygen
c. Nasogastric tube and antibiotics
d. Nasogastric tube and intravenous fluid
e. Nasogastric tube and intravenous fluid and consider caesarean section

9. You (SHO) are seeing a 23-week pregnant patient in the antenatal clinic. She is concerned because about a month ago she went to Bangladesh to see her mother. She has just been informed that her mother has been diagnosed with tuberculosis (TB). The patient is certain that she herself has never been vaccinated against TB.

What is the correct next step?

a. Bronchoscopy and washings
b. Chest X-ray
c. Early morning sputum for MC&S
d. Mantoux test
e. Referral to a respiratory physician

10. You are the SHO working in antenatal clinic and you review a 28-year-old woman who is currently 12 weeks pregnant. You are checking her booking blood and urine results and you note that the midstream urine (MSU) culture has grown *E. coli* >200 colony-forming units per millilitre. She is asymptomatic and therefore reluctant to take any medication. She would like to know the likelihood of her having symptoms and urinary tract infection (UTI) if she is left untreated. Which of the following options is correct?

a. 10% of women will develop symptomatic UTI and 20% acute pyelonephritis
b. 20% of women will develop symptomatic UTI and 10% acute pyelonephritis
c. 30% of women will develop symptomatic UTI and 30% acute pyelonephritis
d. 30% of women will develop symptomatic UTI and 40% acute pyelonephritis
e. 40% of women will develop symptomatic UTI and 30% acute pyelonephritis

11. You are in the antenatal clinic and you see a 12-week pregnant patient in her second pregnancy. She has come to see you as she had developed postnatal depression in her previous pregnancy. She was started on antidepressants by her GP and after 18 months felt well enough to stop them. She would like to know the likelihood of developing the same problem in this pregnancy. Which of the following options is correct?

a. She has a 50%–75% chance of developing postnatal depression again
b. She is unlikely to develop postnatal depression again as she has fully recovered

   c. She is more likely to have a traumatic birth than the national average
   d. She is more likely to miscarry the pregnancy than the national average
   e. She is more likely to have a stillbirth than the national average

12. Which condition gets worse during the puerperium?
   a. Ehlers–Danlos syndrome
   b. Loeys–Dietz syndrome
   c. Marfan syndrome
   d. Pelvic girdle pain
   e. Psoriatic arthritis

13. You are in the antenatal clinic seeing a primigravida at 12 weeks of pregnancy. These are her booking blood results:
- Hb 130 g/L
- WCC 5.4
- Platelets 50
- MCH 33
- MCV 32

Upon questioning her further, she complains that she bruises easily. What is the most likely diagnosis?
   a. Error of sample
   b. Gestational thrombocytopenia
   c. Idiopathic immune thrombocytopenia
   d. Iron deficiency
   e. Vitamin B1 deficiency

14. You are in the diabetic antenatal clinic and you are seeing a 27-week pregnant patient who has just been diagnosed with gestational diabetes, based on a recent glucose tolerance test (GTT). She would like to know what the chances are that she will require medication either orally or injectables, even if she does maintain a good diet and exercise. Which of the following options is correct?
   a. 5%
   b. 15%
   c. 25%
   d. 35%
   e. 45%

15. Which of the following statements is true regarding preexisting diabetes and pregnancy?
   a. All women with preexisting diabetes should be delivered at 37 weeks
   b. All women with preexisting diabetes should have 500 μg of folic acid preconceptually
   c. All women with preexisting diabetes should have 5 mg of folic acid preconceptually
   d. If a woman is on metformin, she should stop it preconceptually
   e. The chances of a macrosomic baby or a stillbirth are the same for women who has preexisting diabetes or develops gestational diabetes

ANSWERS

1. e. ultrasound-guided biopsy for histology

    Ultrasound is the primary method to assess a lump and if cancer is suspected, then mammography is performed with fetal shielding. The tissue diagnosis is made based on histology rather than cytology. The reason being that cytology is inconclusive in pregnant women due to the proliferative changes. The histology is similar to age-matched individuals who are not pregnant. To diagnose breast cancer in a pregnant woman, a chest X-ray and liver ultrasound is conducted. Tumour markers such as CA125, CEA and Ca15-3 are not commonly used as they are not reliable in pregnancy.

    Further reading

    - Royal College of Obstetricians and Gynaecologists (RCOG) Green-top Guideline No. 12. Pregnancy and breast cancer. March 2011.
    - StratOG eLearning. RCOG online learning resource. Maternal medicine: Neoplasia in pregnancy. https://stratog.rcog.org.uk/tutorials/core-knowledge/maternal-medicine/neoplasia-pregnancy

2. b. Can attempt to get pregnant now

    It is advised that women should wait for 12–18 months before attempting to get pregnant after bariatric surgery. This will allow stabilization of the body weight and also correction of any nutritional deficiencies as a result of the surgery.

    Further reading

    - Royal College of Obstetricians and Gynaecologists (RCOG) Green-top Guideline No. 72. Care of Women with Obesity in Pregnancy. November 2018.

3. a. Change antihypertensive, start 75 mg aspirin, aim to keep BP less than <150/100

    Chlorothiazide, ACE inhibitors and angiotensin II receptor blockers (ARBs) are teratogenic and can cause congenital anomalies and therefore they need to be changed to another antihypertensive medication earlier during pregnancy. In pregnant women with chronic hypertension and no target organ damage, the aim is to keep the BP <150/100. If there is target organ damage such as kidney disease, it is recommended to maintain the BP lower than 140/90.

    Further reading

    - National Institute of Health and Care Excellence (NICE). Hypertension in pregnancy diagnosis and management. CG107. August 2010.

4. e. Offer varicella zoster immunoglobulin (VZIG) as soon as possible

    If a pregnant woman has no immunity to Varicella Zoster virus (VZV) and has had a significant exposure to a person who had chicken pox, VZIG should be given as soon as possible, preferably within 10 days of exposure. The patient is then considered infectious from 8 to 28 days after the exposure. If the patient does not get VZIG, they are considered infectious from 8 to 21 days after the exposure (incubation period).

Further reading

- Royal College of Obstetricians and Gynaecologists (RCOG) Green-top Guideline. Chickenpox in pregnancy. No. 13. January 2015.
- StratOG eLearning. RCOG online resource. Maternal medicine-Infectious diseases. https://stratog.rcog.org.uk/tutorials/core-knowledge/maternal-medicine/infectious-diseases

5. b. Levonorgestrel-releasing intrauterine system (LNG-IUS)
   Anti-epileptic medication use and contraception methods

Enzyme-inducing drugs: Carbamazepine, phenytoin, phenobarbital, primidone, oxcarbazepine, topiramate and eslicarbazepine are all enzyme-inducing drugs	
Copper intrauterine devices (IUDs), levonorgestrel-releasing intrauterine system (LNG-IUS) and medroxyprogesterone acetate injections	Are not affected by enzyme-inducing anti-epileptic drugs (AEDs).
Combined hormonal contraception, progestogen-only pills, transdermal contraceptive patches, vaginal contraceptive ring and progestogen-only implants	Are affected by AED Risk of failure of contraception is increased with the use of these methods
Non-enzyme-inducing AEDs: sodium valproate, levetiracetam, gabapentin, vigabatrin, tiagabine and pregabalin	
Non-enzyme-inducing drugs as above	Any form of contraception would be acceptable unless there are other contraindications

Further reading

- Royal College of Obstetricians and Gynaecologists (RCOG) Green-top Guideline. Epilepsy in pregnancy. No. 68. June 2016.
- StratOG eLearning. RCOG online resource. Maternal medicine-Neurological disorders. https://stratog.rcog.org.uk/tutorials/core-knowledge/maternal-medicine/neurological-disorders

6. d. Refer to genitourinary medicine (GUM) physician
   Genital herpes and pregnancy
   There is no evidence that primary genital herpes causes miscarriages in the first trimester. If there is a suspicion of genital herpes during pregnancy, then the patient should be referred to a GUM physician who will confirm the diagnosis using a polymerase chain reaction (PCR) test and will treat accordingly. The treatment is to give Acyclovir 400 mg three times daily, usually for 5 days. It is given orally unless there are clinical symptoms and signs of disseminated HSV in which case it is given intravenously.

   Aciclovir is not licensed in pregnancy but is known to be safe. The GUM physician may also screen for other sexually transmitted diseases.

Further reading

- Royal College of Obstetricians and Gynaecologists (RCOG) Management of Genital Herpes in Pregnancy. October 2014.
- StratOG eLearning. RCOG online learning resource. Maternal medicine-Infectious diseases. https://stratog.rcog.org.uk/tutorials/core-knowledge/maternal-medicine/infectious-diseases

7. b.   20%–40%

The maternal mortality with Eisenmenger's syndrome is 20%–40%. Eisenmenger's syndrome is associated with pulmonary hypertension and consequently increases the mortality risk during pregnancy.

Further reading

- Royal College of Obstetricians and Gynaecologists (RCOG). *Cardiac Disease in Pregnancy*: Good Practice 13. London, UK: RCOG Press, 2011.
- StratOG eLearning. RCOG online resource. Maternal medicine-Cardiac disease. https://stratog.rcog.org.uk/cardiac-disease/cardiac-disease

8. b.   Intravenous fluid and oxygen

The differential diagnosis includes acute pancreatitis and/or acute gastritis as per symptoms. In this scenario, in view of extremely raised amylase, the likely diagnosis is acute pancreatitis.

The question is asking for your initial management, which should be oxygen and intravenous fluid. The fluid prevents systemic complications, and the early oxygen supplementation has been shown to prevent organ failure. Analgesia and antibiotics are essential, but this will be part of the subsequent management. There is nothing in the question to suggest that early delivery is indicated.

Further reading

- Skubic JJ, Salim A. Emergency general surgery in pregnancy. *Trauma Surg Acute Care Open* 2017; 2:1–5.
- StratOG eLearning. RCOG online resource. Maternal medicine - liver and gastrointestinal disease. https://stratog.rcog.org.uk/tutorials/core-knowledge/maternal-medicine/liver-and-gastrointestinal-disease

9. d.   Mantoux test

To diagnose latent TB, the first test that should be done is the Mantoux test. If it is positive, then an interferon-gamma (IFN-γ) release assay should be done on the blood sample. If this test is positive, then the patient should be investigated for active TB with a sputum sample and imaging. The BCG vaccine should not be given in pregnancy as it is a live vaccine.

IFN-γ release assay is a blood test which can aid in diagnosing Mycobacterium tuberculosis infection. However, it does not help to differentiate between latent infections from tubercular disease. This assay helps detection of the secretion of IFN-γ in sampled lymphocytes following stimulation with few (2–3) proteins that are rather specific for *Mycobacterium tuberculosis*.

Further reading

- Goldie MH, Brightling CE. Asthma in pregnancy. *The Obstetrician & Gynaecologist* 2013; 15:241–245.
- StratOG eLearning. RCOG online resource. Maternal medicine - Respiratory disease. https://stratog.rcog.org.uk/tutorials/core-knowledge/maternal-medicine/respiratory-disease

10. e.   40% of women will develop symptomatic UTI and 30% acute pyelonephritis

At 12 weeks gestation, all women are screened for asymptomatic bacteriuria via culture rather than urine dipstick alone. If the culture is positive, treatment is essential as 40% of women will develop symptomatic UTI and 30% acute pyelonephritis. However, despite treatment, 30% of women will have a relapse of bacteriuria; therefore, monthly testing is required after treatment.

Further reading

- McCormick T, Ashe RG, Kearney PM. Urinary tract infection in pregnancy. *The Obstetrician & Gynaecologist* 2008; 10(3):156–162.
- StratOG eLearning. RCOG online resource. Maternal medicine - Renal disease. https://stratog.rcog.org.uk/tutorials/core-knowledge/maternal-medicine/renal-disease

11. a.   She has a 50%–75% chance of developing postnatal depression again

Having had postnatal depression previously, this patient has a 50%–75% chance of developing it again; therefore, one must be aware of early signs of depression, identify and treat early.

Further reading

- National Institute for Health and Care Excellence (NICE). *Antenatal and Postnatal Mental Health: Clinical Management and Service Guidance*: CG192. London, UK: NICE, 2014.
- StratOG eLearning. RCOG online learning resource. Maternal medicine - Perinatal mental health. https://stratog.rcog.org.uk/tutorials/core-knowledge/maternal-medicine/perinatal-mental-health

12. e.   Psoriatic arthritis

Psoriatic arthritis is an autoimmune condition, and the immune response is altered postpartum, therefore it may worsen. The other conditions are connective tissue disorders which are not related to the immunity and therefore unlikely to flare.

Further reading

- Cauldwell M, Nelson-Piercy C. Maternal and fetal complications of systemic lupus erythematosus. *The Obstetrician & Gynaecologist* 2012; 14:167–174.
- StratOG eLearning. RCOG online learning resource. Maternal medicine - connective tissue, bone and joint disorder. https://stratog.rcog.org.uk/tutorials/core-knowledge/maternal-medicine/connective-tissue-bone-and-joint-disorders

13. c. Idiopathic immune thrombocytopenia

The low platelets and her history suggest that she is likely to have idiopathic immune thrombocytopenia. Other signs of idiopathic immune thrombocytopenia are gingivitis, menorrhagia, nose bleeds and petechiae.

Further reading

- Myers B. Thrombocytopenia in pregnancy. *The Obstetrician & Gynaecologist* 2009; 11:177–183.
- StratOG eLearning. RCOG online resource. Maternal medicine - haematological disorders. https://stratog.rcog.org.uk/tutorials/core-knowledge/maternal-medicine/haematological-disorders

14. b. 15%

According to NICE Guideline 63 (Diabetes in pregnancy), 10%–20% of women with gestation diabetes will require some form of medication, despite an adequate diet and exercise. The medication will be either oral hypoglycaemics or insulin therapy. Patients should be informed appropriately.

Further reading

- National Institute for Health and Care Excellence (NICE). *Diabetes in Pregnancy: Management of Diabetes and Its Complications from Pre-conception to the Postnatal Period.* London, UK, March 2008.

15. c. All women with preexisting diabetes should have 5 mg of folic acid preconceptually.

Further reading

- National Institute for Health and Care Excellence (NICE). *Diabetes in Pregnancy: Management of Diabetes and Its Complications from Pre-conception to the Postnatal Period.* London, UK, March 2008.

KNOWLEDGE AREAS 7 AND 8: MANAGEMENT OF LABOUR AND MANAGEMENT OF DELIVERY

QUESTIONS

1. Regarding oxytocin and its analogue Syntocinon, which of the following is false?
   a. Oxytocin is released in the posterior pituitary
   b. Oxytocin stimulates contraction of the myoepithelial cells in the breast
   c. Oxytocin inhibits prolactin secretion
   d. Prolonged exposure to Syntocinon causes downregulation of oxytocin receptors
   e. Prolonged infusion of Syntocinon can cause hyponatraemia

2. With regard to synthesis of adrenal hormones, which of the following is true?
   a. ACTH stimulates aldosterone secretion
   b. Zona reticularis does not synthesize androgens
   c. Zona fasciculata secretes aldosterone
   d. Zona reticularis synthesizes oestrogen precursor
   e. Zona glomerulosa secretes adrenaline

3. You are the labour ward registrar and you have been asked to review a patient. The patient is nulliparous and is currently at 40 weeks gestation. She was at low risk antenatally and is on the labour ward as she requested an epidural. She currently has an epidural in situ and her cervix is fully dilated. She had 2 hours as a passive second stage and has now been pushing for 30 minutes. The midwife examined her and says the fetal head is, in the occipito-anterior (OA), position at station +1 no caput or moulding. The CTG is normal. What is your recommendation?
   a. Caesarean section now
   b. Continue pushing for 30 minutes
   c. Continue pushing for 60 minutes
   d. Instrumental delivery now
   e. Undertake a vaginal examination of the patient yourself

4. You are the labour ward registrar and you have been asked for advice. The patient is multiparous and is currently at 40 weeks gestation. She was at low risk antenatally and is on the labour ward as she has had a previous postpartum haemorrhage. She is fully dilated and is managing to control the pain well with Entonox only. She had 1 hour as a passive stage and has been pushing for 60 minutes. The midwife examined her and says the fetal head is OA, station is +1, no caput or moulding. The CTG is normal. What is your recommendation?
   a. Caesarean section now
   b. Continue pushing for 30 minutes
   c. Continue pushing for 60 minutes
   d. Instrumental delivery now
   e. Undertake a vaginal examination of the patient yourself

5. You are the labour ward registrar and you have been asked for advice. The patient is a para 2 and is currently at 40 weeks gestation. She was at low risk antenatally and is on the labour ward as she requests an epidural. She is now fully dilated and has an epidural in situ. She had 1 hour as a passive stage and has just started pushing. The midwife examined her and says the fetal head is OA, station is +1 (see previous question), no caput or moulding. The CTG is normal. What is your recommendation?
   a. Caesarean section now
   b. Continue pushing for 30 minutes
   c. Continue pushing for 60 minutes
   d. Instrumental delivery now
   e. Undertake a vaginal examination of the patient yourself

6. You are the labour ward registrar and you have been asked for advice. The patient is a para 3 and is currently at 40 weeks gestation. She was at low risk antenatally and is on the labour ward as she has had a previous postpartum haemorrhage. She is fully dilated and is managing to control the pain well with Entonox only. She had 30 minutes as a passive stage and has been pushing for 30 minutes. The midwife examined her and says the fetal head is OA, station is +1 (see previous question), no caput or moulding. The CTG is normal. What is your recommendation?
   a. Caesarean section now
   b. Continue pushing for 30 minutes
   c. Continue pushing for 60 minutes
   d. Instrumental delivery now
   e. Undertake a vaginal examination of the patient yourself

7. You and your registrar have just repaired a 3b perineal tear in a nulliparous patient. The repair went well and there were no complications. Your registrar asks you to prescribe antibiotics for the patient. The patient wants to know the likelihood of the wound being infected. Which of the following options is correct?
   a. 4/100
   b. 5/100

c. 6/100
d. 7/100
e. 8/100

8. You and your registrar have just repaired a 3c perineal tear in a nulliparous patient. The repair went well and there were no complications. The patient wants to know the likelihood of the faecal urgency. Which of the following options is correct?
   a. 16/100
   b. 26/100
   c. 36/100
   d. 46/100
   e. 56/100

9. Regarding adrenocorticotropic hormone (ACTH), which of the following is false?
   a. Secretion is controlled by hypothalamus
   b. Promotes glucose uptake
   c. Mainly promotes cortisol secretion
   d. Promotes release of vasopressin
   e. Levels normally rise throughout pregnancy

10. Which of the following promotes lactation?
    a. High concentration of oestrogen
    b. A rise in progesterone levels
    c. Prolactin
    d. Dopamine
    e. Cabergoline

11. In which of the following is the anion gap not increased?
    a. Alkalosis
    b. Ketoacidosis
    c. Lactic acidosis
    d. Hyperosmolar acidosis
    e. Salicylate poisoning

12. You are in the antenatal clinic and you are reviewing a 17-week pregnant patient who is a para 1 and had normal vaginal delivery previously. Her last baby was admitted to the neonatal unit with early-onset GBS disease and required 7 days of antibiotics. What is your recommendation?
    a. Bacteriological testing should be carried out at 35–37 weeks
    b. Bacteriological testing should be carried out at 30–32 weeks
    c. Give intrapartum antibiotics without undertaking bacteriological testing
    d. No need for bacteriological testing in this pregnancy
    e. No need for antibiotics in this labour

13. Which of the following is false regarding fetal circulation?
    a. The blood in the umbilical vein and ductus venosus is 70%–80% saturated with oxygen

b. Right–left shunt through the foramen ovale is maintained by high venous return from placenta
c. Right–left shunt through the ductus arteriosus is maintained by high pulmonary vascular resistance
d. At birth, the ductus arteriosus closes due to direct effect of increasing PCO_2
e. At birth, the ductus arteriosus closes due to direct effect of increasing PO_2

14. Which of the following is not a tocolytic agent?
    a. Atosiban
    b. Entonox
    c. Nifedipine
    d. Magnesium sulphate
    e. Nitroglycerin

15. Which of the following is caused by oxytocin?
    a. Bradycardia
    b. Hypernatraemia
    c. Dehydration
    d. Neonatal jaundice
    e. Hyperkalaemia

16. Which of the following is an inhaled anaesthetic agent?
    a. Etomidate
    b. Halothane
    c. Ketamine
    d. Isofluratone
    e. Benzocaine

17. With regard to surfactant, which of the following statements is false?
    a. Is synthesized by type 2 pneumocytes
    b. Reduces the surface tension in the alveoli
    c. Increased amounts result in collapse of the lung
    d. Lack or inadequate synthesis in preterm babies results in respiratory distress syndrome (RDS)
    e. Can be given through an endotracheal tube in newborns

18. Which of the following is a contraindication to beta-agonist tocolytic therapy during pregnancy?
    a. Hypothyroidism
    b. Well-controlled diabetes
    c. Mild asthma
    d. History of epilepsy
    e. Severe cardiac disease

ANSWERS

1. c. Oxytocin inhibits prolactin secretion

    Oxytocin is produced in the supraoptic and paraventricular nuclei of the hypothalamus, but it is stored and released by the posterior pituitary. It promotes prolactin secretion and also uterine prostaglandin release.

    Further reading

    - Strat OG: Management of labour and birth.
    - National Institute for Health and Clinical Excellence. *Inducing Labour.* Clinical Guideline 70. London, UK: NICE, 2008.

2. d. Zona reticularis synthesizes oestrogen precursor

    The adrenal gland is divided into outer cortex and inner medulla. The cortex is further divided into three zones: (a) Outer, zona glomerulosa – secretes mineralocorticoids (aldosterone). (b) Middle, zona fasciculata – primarily secretes glucocorticoids, for example, cortisol. (c) Inner, zona reticularis – secretes small quantities of androgens. The outer zone is under the control of the renin–angiotensin system and the middle/inner zones are under the control of ACTH.

    Mnemonic

    G – Zona glomerulosa – mineralocorticoids.

    F – Zona fasciculata – glucocorticoids.

    R – Zona reticularis – androgens.

    Further reading

    - Strat OG Management of labour and birth.
    - Zakar T, Hertelendy F. Progesterone withdrawal: Key to parturition. *American Journal of Obstetrics and Gynecology* 2007; 196:289–296. [Abstract]

3. b. Continue pushing for 30 minutes

4. d. Instrumental delivery now

    It is recommended that nulliparous women, with an epidural, have an instrumental delivery if there is a lack of continuing progress for 3 hours (total of active and passive second-stage labour) or for 2 hours without regional anaesthesia.

    Further reading

    - Royal College of Obstetricians and Gynaecologists (RCOG). Green-top Guideline No. 26. January 2011.
    - National Institute for Health and Care Excellence. *Intrapartum Care for Healthy Women and Babies. Clinical Guideline 190.* London, UK: NICE, 2014.

5. c. Continue pushing for 60 minutes

It is recommended that multiparous women, with an epidural, have an instrumental delivery if there is a lack of continuing progress for 2 hours (total of active and passive second-stage labour) or for 1 hour without regional anaesthesia.

Further reading

- Royal College of Obstetricians and Gynaecologists (RCOG). Green-top Guideline No. 26. January 2011.
- National Institute for Health and Care Excellence. *Intrapartum Care for Healthy Women and Babies. Clinical Guideline 190.* London, UK: NICE, 2014.

6. d. Instrumental delivery now

It is recommended that nulliparous women, with an epidural, have an instrumental delivery if there is a lack of continuing progress for 3 hours (total of active and passive second-stage labour) or for 2 hours without regional anaesthesia.

It is recommended that multiparous women, with an epidural, have an instrumental delivery if there is a lack of continuing progress for 2 hours (total of active and passive second-stage labour) or 1 hour without regional anaesthesia.

Further reading

- Royal College of Obstetricians and Gynaecologists (RCOG). Green-top Guideline No. 26. January 2011.
- National Institute for Health and Care Excellence. *Intrapartum Care for Healthy Women and Babies. Clinical Guideline 190.* London, UK: NICE, 2014.

7. e. 8/100

8 in 100 women will develop an infection and that is why antibiotics are recommended.

Further reading

- Royal College of Obstetricians and Gynaecologists. Consent Advice No. 9 June 2010. Repair of third and fourth degree perineal tears following childbirth.

8. b. 26/100

26% of women will develop faecal incontinence.

Further reading

- Royal College of Obstetricians and Gynaecologists. Consent Advice No. 9 June 2010. Repair of third and fourth degree perineal tears following childbirth.
- Royal College of Obstetricians and Gynaecologists. The OASI Care Bundle Project [Accessed November 2019].

9. d. Promotes release of vasopressin

ACTH is a polypeptide hormone. It is secreted by the pituitary gland (anterior pituitary). It is released in times of biological stress and forms part of the hypothalamo–pituitary–adrenal axis.

Further reading

- Strat OG: Mechanisms of normal labour and birth.

10. c. Prolactin

Breast growth during pregnancy is promoted by oestrogens, progesterones, human placental lactogen and prolactin. A fall in progesterone promotes lactation. Dopamine inhibits prolactin secretion. Cabergoline (dopamine agonist) inhibits prolactin secretion and therefore inhibits lactation.

The lactogenic effect of prolactin and human placental lactogen is normally inhibited by progesterone. Fall in progesterone levels after delivery removes this inhibitory effect and promotes milk secretion.

Further reading

- Strat OG: Mechanisms of normal labour and birth.
- Zakar T, Hertelendy F. Progesterone withdrawal: Key to parturition. *American Journal of Obstetrics and Gynecology* 2007; 196:289–296. [Abstract]

11. a. Alkalosis

Anion gap is also increased in poisoning with ethylene glycol, paraldehyde and methanol, whereas it is decreased with bromide poisoning.

Further reading

- Strat OG: Obstetric analgesia and anaesthesia.
- Alleemudder DI, Kuponiyi Y, Kuponiyi C, McGlennan A, Fountain S, Kasivisvanathan R. Analgesia for labour: An evidence-based insight for the obstetrician. *The Obstetrician & Gynaecologist* 2015; 17:147–155.

12. a. Bacteriological testing should be carried out at 35–37 weeks

If group B streptococcus was found in the last pregnancy, the chances of the patient having it in this pregnancy are 50%. The patient should be offered bacteriological testing between 35 and 37 weeks and treated with intrapartum antibiotics if found to be positive.

Further reading

- Royal College of Obstetricians and Gynaecologists. Prevention of Early-onset Neonatal Group B Streptococcal Disease. Green-top Guideline No. 36.

13. d. At birth, the ductus arteriosus closes due to direct effect of increasing PCO_2

Further reading

- Strat OG: Assessment of fetal wellbeing.

- Sacco A, Muglu J, Navaratnarajah R, Hogg M. ST analysis for intrapartum fetal monitoring. *The Obstetrician & Gynaecologist* 2015; 17:5–12.

14. b. Entonox

Entonox is a combination of 50% oxygen and 50% nitrous oxide. It is used in labour analgesia and is not a tocolytic agent. The other tocolytic agents include ritodrine and terbutaline.

Further reading

- Strat OG: Preterm labour.
- Royal College of Obstetricians and Gynaecologists. *Tocolysis for Women in Preterm Labour: Green-top Guideline 1B*. London, UK: RCOG Press, 2011.

15. d. Neonatal jaundice

Further reading

- Strat OG: Induction of labour and prolonged pregnancy.
- Jozwiak M, Bloemenkamp KWM, Kelly AJ, Mol BWJ, Irion O, Boulvain M. Mechanical methods for induction of labour. *The Cochrane Database of Systematic Reviews* 2012; (3):CD001233.

16. b. Halothane

Etomidate is used intravenously and is not an inhalational anaesthetic agent. Ketamine is used intravenously and is not an inhalational anaesthetic agent. Isofluratone is not a real drug. Bupivacaine is a local anaesthetic agent and is commonly used for epidural analgesia.

Further reading

- Strat OG: Obstetric analgesia and anaesthesia.
- The Association of Anesthetists of Great Britain & Ireland. OAA/AAGBI Guidelines for Obstetric Anaesthetic Services 2013.

17. c. Increased amounts result in collapse of the lung

Type 1 pneumocytes are squamous cells lining the alveoli and they help in gaseous exchange.

Surfactant is synthesized by type 2 pneumocytes in the alveoli. It reduces the surface tension and helps in expansion of the lungs. The inability of the immature lungs to synthesize surfactant in adequate amounts in preterm babies can result in respiratory distress syndrome (RDS).

Further reading

- Strat OG: Assessment of fetal wellbeing.
- Sacco A, Muglu J, Navaratnarajah R, Hogg M. ST analysis for intrapartum fetal monitoring. *The Obstetrician & Gynaecologist* 2015; 17:5–12.

18. e. Severe cardiac disease

Beta-agonists used for tocolysis for preterm labour are non-selective and therefore act on both beta-1 and beta-2 receptors. Beta-2-agonists act on the receptors located on the myocytes and initiate myometrial relaxation by stimulation of cAMP (cyclic adenomonophosphate). This reduces the calcium influx along with inhibition of the myosin light chain kinase. Examples are ritodrine, salbutamol and terbutaline.

The side effects are tremor, palpitations, headache, tachycardia and serious complications such as pulmonary oedema. Beta-receptor stimulation also leads to vasodilatation and as a result there is a compensatory tachycardia, increase in stroke volume and increase in the cardiac output.

Stimulation of beta-2 receptors causes glycogenolysis and elevation in the blood sugar levels, while beta-1-receptor stimulation causes mobilization of free fatty acids and glycolysis. The aforementioned actions explain the indications for contraindications.

On the other hand, the calcium channel blocker nifedipine inhibits the calcium influx across the cell membranes and therefore reduces the tone of the smooth muscle cells in the uterus.

Further reading

- Strat OG: Preterm labour.
- Royal College of Obstetricians and Gynaecologists. *Tocolysis for Women in Preterm Labour: Green-top Guideline 1B.* London, UK: RCOG Press, 2011.

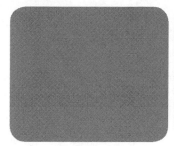

KNOWLEDGE AREA 9: POSTPARTUM PROBLEMS

QUESTIONS

1. Which of the following is true regarding prolactin?
   a. Is a dipeptide
   b. Is evolutionarily not related to growth hormone
   c. Is structurally related to thyroid hormone
   d. Is structurally related to growth hormone
   e. High levels promote pulsatile GnRH secretion

2. Which of the following does not promote prolactin secretion?
   a. Vasopressin
   b. Oxytocin
   c. Dopamine
   d. Vasoactive intestinal peptide
   e. Thyrotropin-releasing hormone

3. Which of the following is a physiological cause for raised prolactin?
   a. Chronic renal failure
   b. Herpes zoster infection
   c. Pituitary adenoma
   d. Sexual intercourse
   e. Use of haloperidol

4. Which of the following promotes lactation?
   a. High concentration of oestrogen
   b. High progesterone levels
   c. Prolactin
   d. Dopamine
   e. Cabergoline

5. You are seeing reviewing a patient on the postnatal ward who is now para 1 after having a Caesarean section the previous day for failure to progress at 6 cm. She is trying to breastfeed and would like advice about contraception. She thinks she will forget to take pills and does not like injections.
   Which of the following would you advise?
   a. Combined hormonal contraception
   b. Depot medroxyprogesterone acetate

   c. Levonorgestrel-releasing intrauterine system

   d. Progesterone only pill

   e. Progesterone only implant

6. You are seeing reviewing a patient on the postnatal ward who is now para 1 after having a Caesarean section 5 days ago for failure to progress at 6 cm. She is breastfeeding and would like advice about contraception. She thinks she will forget to take pills.

     Which of the following would you advise?

   a. Combined hormonal contraception

   b. Depot medroxyprogesterone acetate

   c. Levonorgestrel-releasing intrauterine system

   d. Progesterone only pill

   e. Progesterone only implant

7. You are called by the community midwife for some advice. She is seeing reviewing a para 1 patient who had a normal vaginal delivery 25 days ago. She has just seen her general practitioner (GP) who has inserted a progesterone-only implant. The patient is asking if she needs additional contraceptive precautions since the insertion of the implant. The patient is not breastfeeding and had no past medical history.

     What would your advice be?

   a. No additional contraceptive precautions required

   b. 2 days of additional contraceptive precautions required since the insertion of the implant

   c. 5 days of additional contraceptive precautions required since the insertion of the implant

   d. 7 days of additional contraceptive precautions required since the insertion of the implant

   e. 9 days of additional contraceptive precautions required since the insertion of the implant

8. You are the doctor on call in charge of gynaecological emergencies. You have been called by the GP for some advice about a patient who had normal vaginal delivery 19 days ago. It was an uncomplicated pregnancy and delivery. The patient had unprotected intercourse the previous night and is now worried about getting pregnant.

     What is your advice regarding contraception?

   a. Copper intrauterine device

   b. No contraception required

   c. Levonorgestrel 1.5 mg

   d. Levonorgestrel 3 mg

   e. Ulipristal acetate 30 mg

9. You are seeing reviewing a 35-year-old patient in maternity triage. She had an uncomplicated pregnancy and normal vaginal delivery 5 days ago. Her husband brought her in because he was worried. She is crying a lot, is irritable all the time and says she is anxious.

   What is your advice?
   a. Admit to the postnatal ward
   b. Admit to a mother–baby unit
   c. Refer to local psychology services
   d. Reassure and monitor
   e. Start antidepressants

10. You are seeing reviewing a 35-year-old patient in maternity triage. She had an uncomplicated pregnancy and normal vaginal delivery 10 days ago. Her husband brought her in as he was worried because she has not eaten for the last 4 days, has not showered for the last 8 days, shows little interest in the baby and feels persistently low in mood. What is your advice?
    a. Admit to the postnatal ward
    b. Admit to a mother–baby unit
    c. Refer to local psychology services
    d. Reassure and monitor
    e. Start antidepressants

11. According to the UK Centre for Maternal and Child Enquiries Survey 2005–2008, which of the following is *not* a risk factor for maternal sepsis?
    a. Anaemia
    b. Black or minority ethnic group origin
    c. Cervical cerclage
    d. Impaired glucose tolerance/diabetes
    e. Low BMI

12. Regarding endotoxin, which of the following is *true*:
    a. Is a protein substance
    b. Is heat labile
    c. Activates macrophages to release interleukins
    d. Can be modified by chemicals to produce a toxoid
    e. Is secreted by bacterial cells

13. You are the SHO in charge of labour ward. You are asked to see a patient who was referred to you by the GP as she was feeling "unwell." She had a Caesarean section 5 days ago and was discharged on day 1, with no complications. She had an uneventful pregnancy but had a Caesarean section due to presumed fetal distress. In maternity triage, her temperature is 39°, respiratory rate 30 and her pulse 112 beats per minute (bpm). Which of the following is the most important initial investigation?
    a. Blood cultures
    b. High vaginal swab
    c. Lactate
    d. Low vaginal swab
    e. Urine cultures

ANSWERS

1. d. Is structurally related to growth hormone

    Prolactin is a polypeptide. Prolactin is evolutionarily structurally related to growth hormone. High levels of prolactin inhibit pulsatile GnRH secretion.

    Further reading

    - Sarris I, Sangeeta A, Susan B. *Training in Obstetrics and Gynaecology: The Essential Curriculum.* Oxford, UK: Oxford University Press, 2009, pp. 394–395.

2. c. Dopamine

    Dopamine inhibits prolactin secretion. Thyrotropin-releasing hormone (TRH) also promotes prolactin secretion.

    Further reading

    - Sarris I, Sangeeta A, Susan B. *Training in Obstetrics and Gynaecology: The Essential Curriculum.* Oxford, UK: Oxford University Press, 2009, pp. 394–395.

3. d. The physiological causes of raised prolactin include pregnancy, lactation, breast stimulation, stress, sexual intercourse and exercise. The pathological causes of increase in prolactin levels are pituitary adenomas (micro- and macroprolactinomas), polycystic ovarian syndrome (PCOS), chronic renal failure, herpes zoster pain, drugs (phenothiazines, haloperidol, metoclopramide, methyldopa, morphine, methadone, oestrogens, cocaine and cimetidine).

    Further reading

    - Sarris I, Sangeeta A, Bewley Susan B. *Training in Obstetrics and Gynaecology: The Essential Curriculum.* Oxford, UK: Oxford University Press, 2009, pp. 394–395.

4. c. Prolactin

    Breast growth during pregnancy is promoted by oestrogens, progesterones, human placental lactogen and prolactin. Dopamine inhibits prolactin secretion. Cabergoline (dopamine agonist) inhibits prolactin secretion and therefore inhibits lactation.

    The lactogenic effect of prolactin and human placental lactogen is normally inhibited by progesterone. Fall in progesterone levels after delivery removes this inhibitory effect and promotes milk secretion.

    Further reading

    - Sarris I, Sangeeta A, Bewley Susan B. *Training in Obstetrics and Gynaecology: The Essential Curriculum.* Oxford, UK: Oxford University Press, 2009, pp. 394–395.

5. c.   Levonorgestrel-releasing intrauterine system
        Levonorgestrel-releasing intrauterine system can be inserted within
        48 hours of delivery whether the patient is breastfeeding or not. There is
        limited evidence of the use of an intrauterine device from 48 hours to
        4 weeks, and therefore the recommendation is to insert it within 48 hours.

Further reading

- FSRH UK Medical Eligibility Criteria for Contraceptive use - UKMEC.
  https://www.fsrh.org/ukmec/
- Sarris I, Sangeeta A, Susan B. *Training in Obstetrics and Gynaecology:
  The Essential Curriculum.* Oxford, UK: Oxford University Press, 2009,
  pp. 394–395.

6. e.   Progesterone-only implant
        The combined hormonal contraception is contraindicated at less
        than 4 weeks. Depot medroxyprogesterone acetate is rated as 2 under
        UKMEC. There is limited evidence of the use of an intrauterine device
        from 48 hours to 4 weeks, thus leaving progesterone-only implant as the
        only option.

Further reading

- FSRH UK Medical Eligibility Criteria for Contraceptive use - UKMEC.
  https://www.fsrh.org/ukmec/
- Sarris I, Sangeeta A, Susan B. *Training in Obstetrics and Gynaecology:
  The Essential Curriculum.* Oxford, UK: Oxford University Press, 2009,
  pp. 394–395.

7. d.   7 days of additional contraceptive precautions required since the insertion
        of the implant
        If the progesterone-only implant was inserted before day
        21 postpartum, no additional days would be required. However, as
        this was inserted after 21 days, then 7 days of additional contraceptive
        precautions is required.

Further reading

- FSRH UK Medical Eligibility Criteria for Contraceptive use - UKMEC.
  https://www.fsrh.org/ukmec/

8. b.   No contraception required
        Emergency contraception is not indicated if unprotected intercourse
        occurred after 21 days of delivery.

Further reading

- FSRH UK Medical Eligibility Criteria for Contraceptive use - UKMEC.
  https://www.fsrh.org/ukmec/
- Sarris I, Sangeeta A, Susan B. *Training in Obstetrics and Gynaecology:
  The Essential Curriculum.* Oxford, UK: Oxford University Press, 2009,
  pp. 394–395.

9. d.   Reassure and monitor

This patient has postnatal blues. It usually occurs between day 3 and 10, but peaks on day 5 and lasts 48 hours. It is common and affects 50%–80% of women. The symptoms are self-limiting and resolve with reassurance.

Further reading

● RCOG online learning resource: StratOG: Postpartum and Neonatal problems. https://elearning.rcog.org.uk/tutorials/core-training/postpartum-and-neonatal-problems

10. c.   Refer to local psychology services

This patient has mild postnatal depression. Postnatal depression affects 10–15 in every 100 women. There is a gradual onset of symptoms in the first 2 weeks after birth, and then they peak at 2–4 weeks and 10–14 weeks after birth. As this patient has mild depression, she should be referred to local psychology services. The services will give her reading plus online material that she can read, based on a cognitive behavioural model. It is a 9–12-week course with 8 face-to-face or telephone conversations.

Further reading

● RCOG online learning resource: StratOG: Postpartum and Neonatal problems. https://elearning.rcog.org.uk/tutorials/core-training/postpartum-and-neonatal-problems

11. e.   Low BMI

Obesity is a risk factor for sepsis, not low BMI. Other risk factors include immunosuppressant medication, vaginal discharge, history of pelvic infection, amniocentesis and other invasive procedures, cervical cerclage, prolonged spontaneous rupture of membranes, vaginal trauma, caesarean section, wound haematoma, retained products of conception and Group A *Streptococcus* infection in close contacts/family members.

Further reading

● Royal College of Obstetricians and Gynaecologist (RCOG). Green-top Guideline No. 64b. Bacterial Sepsis following Sepsis. April 2012.
● Centre for Maternal and Child Enquiries (CMACE). Saving Mothers' Lives: Reviewing maternal deaths to make motherhood safer: 2006–2008. The Eighth Report on Confidential Enquiries into Maternal Deaths in the United Kingdom. *BJOG* 2011; 118 Suppl 1:1–203.

12. c.   Activates macrophages to release interleukins

Endotoxin (lipopolysaccharide) is part of the outer membrane of Gram-negative organisms. It is heat stable (cannot be modified by either heat or chemicals). It is not strongly immunogenic and therefore not convertible to a toxoid, unlike exotoxins (can be modified by heat or chemicals to form toxoid and can be used as a vaccine). Endotoxins activate macrophages and promote release of TNF-α and interleukin-1 and interleukin-6. This leads to tissue damage.

Exotoxins are protein substances and secreted by certain bacterial Gram-negative and Gram-positive organisms. These substances are responsible for lysis of cells by damaging cell membranes.

Further reading

● Sarris I, Sangeeta A, Susan B. *Training in Obstetrics and Gynaecology: The Essential Curriculum.* Oxford, UK: Oxford University Press, 2009, pp. 394–395.

13. c. Lactate

This patient is septic and needs treatment and investigations immediately and simultaneously. The lactate should be done within 1 hour of arrival.

Further reading

● RCOG online learning resource: STratOG: Postpartum and Neonatal problems. https://elearning.rcog.org.uk/tutorials/core-training/postpartum-and-neonatal-problems

KNOWLEDGE AREA 10: GYNAECOLOGICAL PROBLEMS

QUESTIONS

1. With regard to development of secondary sexual characteristics (males and females), which of the following is false?
   a. Breast growth in females usually begins between 9 and 13 years of age
   b. Breast development occurs in three stages
   c. Increase in the size of testes is the first sign of puberty in boys
   d. The growth spurt in boys usually starts 12 months after the increase in the testicular volume
   e. The appearance of pubic hair follows the appearance of breast buds in females

2. You are in the gynaecology clinic and you have been asked to review a 17-year-old patient with primary amenorrhoea. She has normal secondary sexual characteristics and her external genitalia appear normal. She also complains of a swelling in her right groin. What is the diagnosis?
   a. Androgen insensitivity syndrome
   b. Congenital adrenal hyperplasia
   c. Klinefelter syndrome
   d. Rokitansky syndrome
   e. Turner syndrome

3. You are in the gynaecology clinic and you have been asked to review a 17-year-old patient with primary amenorrhoea. She has normal secondary sexual characteristics and her external genitalia appear normal. An ultrasound reveals small ovaries and absent uterus. What is the diagnosis?
   a. Androgen insensitivity syndrome
   b. Congenital adrenal hyperplasia
   c. Klinefelter syndrome
   d. Rokitansky syndrome
   e. Turner syndrome

4. With respect to androgen production in females, which of the following is false?
   a. They are produced by both ovaries and adrenal gland
   b. DHEA is mainly derived from the adrenal gland
   c. Two-thirds of the daily testosterone production is of adrenal origin

    d.   Androgens are mainly excreted as 17-oxosteroids after metabolism

    e.   Androgens exert their effect by binding to intracellular receptors

5. With regard to gonadotropins (FSH and LH), which of the following is false?
   a. The half-life of luteinizing hormone (LH) is 90 minutes
   b. LH has a shorter half-life than FSH
   c. The half-life of FSH is twice that of LH
   d. Less frequent pulses cause no change in the LH and increase in the FSH
   e. FSH and LH are released every 60 minutes during the follicular phase

6. You are in the gynaecology clinic and you are about to review a 35-year-old nulliparous woman who is complaining of severe premenstrual syndrome. She has tried cognitive behaviour therapy (CBT) but it has not worked. She wants to know what the next treatment plan will be.
   a. Combined oral contraceptive
   b. Implanon
   c. Progesterone-only pill
   d. Mirena coil
   e. Selective serotonin reuptake inhibitor (SSRI)

7. You are seeing a 57-year-old woman in the gynaecology clinic. She presented with a history of postmenopausal bleeding (PMB) 2 weeks ago. An ultrasound was arranged and it revealed the endometrial thickness to be 7 mm. Her bleeding has settled now. She has taken tamoxifen in the past for breast cancer. What is the correct next step in her management?
   a. CT
   b. Hysteroscopy and endometrial biopsy
   c. MRI
   d. Repeat ultrasound in 3 months
   e. Repeat ultrasound in 4 months

8. Regarding *Chlamydia trachomatis*, which of the following is false?
   a. Is a facultative intracellular bacterium
   b. Is causative organism for lymphogranuloma venereum
   c. Is the commonest cause of non-gonococcal urethritis in men
   d. Is the most common cause of PID in women
   e. Can cause pneumonia in neonate

9. You are in the sexual health clinic and a 25-year-old patient attends complaining of a green vaginal discharge associated with itching. You perform a Wet-mount microscopy and find motile protozoan. What is the correct treatment?
   a. Amikacin
   b. Azithromycin
   c. Co-amoxiclave
   d. Gentamicin
   e. Metronidazole

10. You are in the sexual health clinic and a 25-year-old patient attends complaining of fishy smelling vaginal discharge, especially after having sexual intercourse. You perform a wet mount microscopy and find clue cells. What is the correct treatment?
    a. Amikacin
    b. Azithromycin
    c. Co-amoxiclav
    d. Gentamicin
    e. Metronidazole

11. Regarding the starting time of the combined oral contraceptive pill, which of the following statements is correct?
    a. First day of menstruation
    b. Seventh day after induced early abortion
    c. Tenth day after delivery in non-lactating woman
    d. 1 month after molar pregnancy
    e. Tenth day after induced late abortion

12. You are seeing a 49-year-old patient in the gynaecology clinic. She had a history of heavy menstrual bleeding, and therefore a mirena intrauterine contraception system was inserted. She was amenorrhoeic for 1.5 years and then started developing heavy periods again. She has had an endometrial biopsy performed which showed endometrial hyperplasia with atypia. What is the correct management?
    a. Insert a new mirena coil
    b. Repeat histology in 4 months
    c. Total abdominal hysterectomy and bilateral salpingo-oophorectomy
    d. Tranexamic acid
    e. Ultrasound in 4 months

13. You are in the gynaecology clinic and you are about to see a 49-year-old woman who would like try hormone replacement therapy, as she is finding the hot flushes difficult to manage. She has no past medical or surgical history. Her last menstrual period was 3 weeks ago. What is the best treatment for her?
    a. Continuous combined HRT
    b. Oestrogen-only pill
    c. Oestrogen-only patch
    d. Sequential combined HRT
    e. Tibolone

14. You are in the gynaecology clinic and you are about to review a 61-year-old woman who would like to consider hormone replacement therapy, as she is finding the hot flushes difficult to manage. She has no past medical or surgical history. She has been amenorrhoeic for the last 18 months. What is the best treatment for her?
    a. Oestrogen-only pill
    b. Oestrogen-only patch

c. Short course of continuous combined HRT

d. Short course of sequential combined HRT

e. Tibolone

15. You are in the gynaecology clinic and you are about to review a 53-year-old woman who would like to consider hormone replacement therapy, as she is finding her hot flushes difficult to manage. She does not have any other symptoms. She had a hysterectomy 7 years ago for fibroids. What is the best treatment for her?

a. Continuous combined HRT

b. Oestrogen-only pill

c. Oestrogen-only patch

d. Sequential combined HRT

e. Tibolone

ANSWERS

1. b. Breast development occurs in three stages

In females, usually breast growth and growth spurt occur first. This is followed by the appearance of axillary hair and then menstruation. Breast development occurs in five stages. The growth spurt in boys usually starts 12 months after increase in the testicular volume.

Further reading

- RCOG online learning resource. StratOG Paediatric and adolescent gynaecology. https://elearning.rcog.org.uk/tutorials/core-knowledge/gynaecological-problems-and-early-pregnancy-loss/paediatric-and-adolescent
- Shayya R, Chang RJ. Reproductive endocrinology of adolescent polycystic ovary syndrome. *BJOG* 2010; 117:150–155.

2. a. Androgen insensitivity syndrome

Androgen insensitivity syndrome (AIS) is a rare condition and is genotypically XY (affects development of child's genitalia and reproductive system)	
Reason for development of female genitalia	The lack of responsiveness of the genitalia to androgens in the fetus prevents or impairs masculinization of the male genitalia but does not impair development of female genital system
Genotype-46 XY	Phenotype: female The patient has normal physical secondary characteristic but a blind ending vaginal end The swelling in the right groin is most likely a testicle, and is usually found in the inguinal canal
AIS can be partial or complete	
Partial AIS	• Partial AIS can include failure of one or both testes to descend after birth into the scrotum. Also these people can have hypospadias (opening of urethra on the underside of the penis) • In this case, there is some effect of testosterone on the genitalia, so the genitalia look between male and female
Complete AIS	• Complete AIS is not obvious at birth. These babies are usually raised as girls as they have a vagina and also labia, although internally they have gonads (testes). There is lack of uterus, cervix, ovaries and fallopian tube • They have well-developed breasts • In this case the testosterone has no effect on the genitalia; therefore, female phenotype

(Continued)

Complete AIS	• There is increased risk of gonadal tumours (germ cell tumours 3.6% at 25 years and 33% at 50 years) developing in the abnormally placed testes (with Y chromosome) in adulthood if gonadectomy is not performed • The incidence of malignancy is low prior to puberty • Therefore, it is recommended that gonads are removed around the time of puberty or just after puberty to help in the full development of secondary sexual characteristics

Clinical presentation:
Lack of menstrual period at puberty or presentation with inguinal hernia premenarche.
If this is partial AIS, intersex problems, gender identity problems and psychological issues
Signs:
Sparse axillary and pubic hair, longer hands and limbs, large feet, nil or minimal acne

Further reading

- https://en.wikipedia.org/wiki/Complete_androgen_insensitivity_syndrome
- RCOG online learning resource. StratOG Paediatric and adolescent gynaecology. https://elearning.rcog.org.uk/tutorials/core-knowledge/gynaecological-problems-and-early-pregnancy-loss/paediatric-and-adolescent
- Shaw R, Luesley D, Monga A. *Gynaecology.* 4th ed. London, UK: Churchill Livingstone, 2010.
- Jeffery E, Kayani S, Garden A. Management of menstrual problems in adolescents with learning and physical disabilities. *The Obstetrician & Gynaecologist* 2013; 15:106–112.

3. d. Rokitansky syndrome
There are normal secondary sexual characteristics but an absent uterus. Surrogacy would be the only option for pregnancy.

Further reading

- Shaw R, Luesley D, Monga A. *Gynaecology.* 4th ed. London, UK: Churchill Livingstone, 2010.
- Tirumuru SS, Arya P, Latthe P. Understanding precocious puberty in girls. *The Obstetrician & Gynaecologist* 2012; 14:121–129.

4. c. Two-thirds of the daily testosterone production is of adrenal origin
Two-thirds of the daily female testosterone production is of ovarian origin.

Further reading

- Parker MA, Sneddon AE, Arbon P. The menstrual disorder of teenagers (MDOT) study: Determining typical menstrual patterns and menstrual disturbance in a large population-based study of Australian teenagers. *BJOG* 2010; 117:185–192.

5. a. The half-life of luteinizing hormone (LH) is 90 minutes

The half-life of the LH is 20 minutes. The gonadotropins are metabolized in the liver and kidneys. The half-life of LH is 20 minutes. FSH and LH levels are high during menstruation and tend to fall during the luteal phase of the cycle. Oestrogen exerts both positive and negative feedback (mediated mainly through the pituitary). Frequent pulses of GnRH cause diminished gonadotropin response (mainly seen in early puberty).

Further reading

- Michala L, Creighton SM. The XY Female. *Best Practice & Research Clinical Obstetrics & Gynaecology* 2010; 24:139–148.

6. e. Selective Serotonin reuptake inhibitor (SSRI)

First-line therapy is exercise and CBT. If that does not work, then continuous or luteal-phase low-dose SSRI should be given.

Further reading

- Royal College of Obstetricians and Gynaecologists. *Management of Premenstrual Syndrome: Green-top Guideline 48*. London, UK: RCOG, 2007.
- Green LJ, O'Brien PMS, Panay N, Craig M. On behalf of the Royal College of Obstetricians and Gynaecologists management of premenstrual syndrome. *BJOG* 2016; doi: 10.1111/1471-0528.14260.

7. b. Hysteroscopy and endometrial biopsy

This patient has a thickened endometrium with a history of PMB, and therefore needs hysteroscopy and endometrial biopsy. Tamoxifen is a selective oestrogen receptor modulator (SERM). Tamoxifen can cause endometrial hyperplasia, the formation of polyps, uterine sarcoma and invasive carcinoma. The risk of endometrial cancer is two- to threefolds greater in women taking tamoxifen than in the general population.

Further reading

- RCOG online learning resource. StratOG. Abnormal uterine bleeding. https://elearning.rcog.org.uk/abnormal-uterine-bleeding/menstrual-cycle/abnormal-uterine-bleeding
- Cooper NAM, Clark TJ. Ambulatory hysteroscopy. *The Obstetrician & Gynaecologist* 2013; 15:159–166.

8. a. Is a facultative intracellular bacterium

It is an obligate intracellular pathogen and cannot grow outside a living cell. *Chlamydia* infection is a sexually transmitted infection. Certain strains of *C. trachomatis* (serovars A, B, Ba, C) are associated with trachoma, which is a major cause of blindness worldwide. Serovars L1, L2 and L3 are associated with lymphogranuloma venereum. Serovars D to K cause non-specific urethritis and epididymitis in men and peri-hepatitis, cervicitis, urethritis, endometritis and salpingitis (infection of upper genital tract leading to PID) in women. It can cause Reiter's syndrome in both men and women (conjunctivitis, proctitis, urethritis and reactive seronegative arthritis). Its long-term sequelae include chronic pelvic pain, infertility and ectopic pregnancy. It is associated with increased rates of transmission of HIV infection. It can be transmitted to the neonate during its passage through the birth canal and may cause conjunctivitis and pneumonia.

The incubation period is 1–3 weeks and men present with mucopurulent urethral discharge (urethritis) and women present with vaginal discharge (cervicitis). Asymptomatic infection is not uncommon in both men and women. Cervical or urethral swabs (first sample of urine in men) are collected for culture and nucleic acid amplification test. It is sensitive to doxycycline and erythromycin group of drugs.

Further reading

- RCOG online learning resource. StratOG. Sexually transmitted infections (Including HIV). https://elearning.rcog.org.uk/ tutorials/core-knowledge/sexual-and-reproductive-health/ sexually-transmitted-infections-including
- Nwokolo NC, Dragovic B, Patel S, Tong CYW, Barker G, Radcliffe K. 2015. UK national guideline for the management of infection with chlamydia trachomatis. *International Journal of STD & AIDS* 2016; 27:251–267.

9. e.   Metronidazole

Trichomonas vaginalis (TV) is a single-celled, flagellated, motile protozoan. It is slightly larger than a granulocyte and depends on adherence to the host cell for its survival. Women can present with yellowish-green frothy vaginal discharge (has odour), itching of the genital area, dysuria and dyspareunia (vaginitis, cervicitis and urethritis). It may lead to premature rupture of membranes and preterm delivery. It can coexist with other genital infections such as gonorrhoea, *Chlamydia* and bacterial vaginosis. Most men are usually asymptomatic and can (rarely) develop genital irritation, epididymitis and prostatitis.

On speculum examination, the vaginal mucosa is erythematous and the cervix is inflamed with numerous petechiae (strawberry appearance). Motile organisms are seen on wet mount saline preparation under the microscope. Wet mount microscopy and cultures are the gold standard for its diagnosis. Metronidazole is the drug of choice for treatment.

Further reading

- RCOG online learning resource. StratOG. Sexually transmitted infections (Including HIV). https://elearning.rcog.org.uk/ tutorials/core-knowledge/sexual-and-reproductive-health/ sexually-transmitted-infections-including
- Sherrard J, Ison C, Moody J, Wainwright E, Wilson J, Sullivan A. United Kingdom national guideline on the management of trichomonas vaginalis. *International Journal of STD & AIDS* 2014; 25:541–549.

10. e. Metronidazole

Bacterial vaginosis (BV) is a polymicrobial superficial vaginal infection due to an overgrowth of anaerobes and is the most common cause of vaginal discharge. *Gardnerella vaginalis* (also known as *Haemophilus vaginalis*) is a facultative, anaerobic, non-flagellated, non-spore-forming bacterium. It is recognized as one of the organisms responsible for causing bacterial vaginosis. The other organisms involved in this pathology are *Bacteroides, Peptostreptococcus, Fusobacterium, Mycoplasma hominis, Mobiluncus* and *Veillonella*.

Women present with thin grey homogeneous vaginal discharge and a characteristic fishy odour (alkalinity of semen may cause a release of volatile amines from the vaginal discharge – forms the basis for the whiff test). The fishy smell is mainly recognized after sexual intercourse. Vulval itching, dysuria and dyspareunia are rare. It is also known to cause vault infection following hysterectomy and pelvic infection after abortion. In pregnant women, it has been associated with premature rupture of membranes and preterm delivery. The following are recognized as risk factors for the development of BV: vaginal douching, antibiotic use, decrease in oestrogen production, presence of intrauterine device and increase in number of sexual partners.

There is an increase in vaginal pH as it is associated with a decrease in lactobacilli (responsible for maintaining the acidic pH) in the vagina. Wet mount saline preparation with vaginal discharge shows clue cells (vaginal epithelial cells have a stippled appearance due to adherence of coccobacilli) under low- and high-power microscopy. The drug used for treatment is metronidazole (single dose of 2 g or 7-day course of oral dose – 500 mg bd for 7 days). Metronidazole is contraindicated during early pregnancy. Topical clindamycin and metronidazole are also useful in returning the vaginal flora to normal.

Amsel's criteria for diagnosis of bacterial vaginosis are (a) thin white homogeneous discharge; (b) increase in vaginal pH (4.5); (c) clue cells on microscopy and (d) whiff test – when a few drops of alkali (10% KOH) are added to vaginal secretions, a fishy smell is released. At least three of the four criteria should be present to make the diagnosis.

Further reading

- RCOG online learning resource. StratOG. Sexually transmitted infections (Including HIV). https://elearning.rcog.org.uk/ tutorials/core-knowledge/sexual-and-reproductive-health/ sexually-transmitted-infections-including
- British Association for Sexual Health and HIV, Clinical Effectiveness Group. *UK National Guideline for the Management of Bacterial Vaginosis 2012.* BASHH, 2012.

11. a. First day of menstruation

Post-abortion, combined pills are started the same or next day, on postnatal day 21 in non-lactating women and should be avoided after a molar pregnancy.

Further reading

- Faculty of Sexual and Reproductive Healthcare. *UK Medical Eligibility Criteria for Contraceptive Use.* London, UK: FSRH, 2016.
- Carey MS, Allen RH. Non-contraceptive uses and benefits of combined oral contraception. *The Obstetrician & Gynaecologist* 2012; 14:223–228.

12. c.   Total abdominal hysterectomy and bilateral salpingo-oophorectomy
Complex hyperplasia with atypia progresses to endometrial cancer in 29%, over 4.1 years.

Further reading

- RCOG online learning resource. StratOG. Abnormal uterine bleeding. https://elearning.rcog.org.uk/abnormal-uterine-bleeding/menstrual-cycle/abnormal-uterine-bleeding
- National Institute for Health and Clinical Excellence. *Heavy Menstrual Bleeding. CG44.* Manchester, UK: NICE, 2007.

13. d.   Sequential combined HRT
If a patient still has periods, then the HRT that she is given should be sequential combined HRT. This is daily oestrogen with the addition of progesterone for 10–12 days in the 28-day cycle. This treatment will ensure that the patient continues to have a monthly withdrawal bleed.

Further reading

- RCOG online learning resource. StratOG. Management of climacteric problems. https://elearning.rcog.org.uk/tutorials/core-knowledge/gynaecological-problems-and-early-pregnancy-loss/management-climacteric
- National Institute for Health and Clinical Excellence. *Menopause: Diagnosis and Management: CG23.* NICE, 2015. www.nice.org.uk

14. c.   Short course of combined HRT
If a patient has been amenorrhoeic for at least 12 months, then she should be given continuous combined HRT. This is oestrogen and progesterone together every day. Initially the patient may have some spotting or a light bleed but this will settle.

In younger women, the risk profile of combined HRT is similar to that of tibolone but for women after 60 years of age, the risks outweigh benefits with tibolone in view of increased risk of stroke with tibolone.

Further reading

- RCOG online learning resource. StratOG. Management of climacteric problems. https://elearning.rcog.org.uk/tutorials/core-knowledge/gynaecological-problems-and-early-pregnancy-loss/management-climacteric
- Tibolone: Risks benefit balance. https://www.gov.uk/drug-safety-update/tibolone-benefit-risk-balance
- National Institute for Health and Clinical Excellence. *Menopause: Diagnosis and Management: CG23.* NICE, 2015.

15. c. Oestrogen-only patch

As the patient has had a total hysterectomy, she only needs oestrogen. The patch is ideal as the side effects are less, and easier to remember.

The use of tibolone would be of value on women who has reduced or loss of libido. The sexual function improvement seems to be increased with the use of tibolone than achieved with conventional hormone replacement therapy. Low or loss of libido and mood problems can be an indication for the use of tibolone if there are no medical contraindications.

Further reading

- RCOG online learning resource. StratOG. Management of climacteric problems. https://elearning.rcog.org.uk/tutorials/core-knowledge/gynaecological-problems-and-early-pregnancy-loss/management-climacteric
- National Institute for Health and Clinical Excellence. *Menopause: Diagnosis and Management. CG23.* NICE, 2015. http://www.nice.org.uk
- Davis, SR. The effects of tibolone on mood and libido. *Menopause* 2002; 9(3):162–170.

QUESTIONS

1. Subfertility is defined as an unwanted delay in conception after 1 year of regular unprotected intercourse. Approximately what percentage of the population will experience subfertility?
   a. 5%
   b. 10%
   c. 15%
   d. 20%
   e. 25%

2. A 32-year-old male teacher presents with his wife to your fertility clinic; they have been trying to have a child for the last 1 year.
      His sperm report is as follows:
   - Volume: 4 mL
   - Total sperm count: 17 million
   - Sperm concentration: 8 million/mL
   - pH: >7.2
   - Overall motility: 10%
   - Normal forms: 3%
   - Vitality: 25%

      What is the diagnosis?
   a. Asthenospermia
   b. Oligozoospermia
   c. Oligoteratozoospermia
   d. Oligoasthenoteratozoospermia
   e. Teratozoospermia

3. You are in clinic, and you are about to see a 28-year-old couple who have been trying to conceive for the last 2 years, primary infertility. The female patient has no past medical history, and all her investigations have been normal. Her male partner had mumps as a teenager. He smokes five cigarettes a day and drinks socially. His results have shown high FSH and LH levels and low

testosterone. His semen analysis shows azoospermia. His karyotyping is normal. What is the correct treatment?
a. Antioxidant treatment for 3 months for the male partner
b. Donor insemination
c. hCG treatment for 6 months for the male partner
d. Male partner to stop smoking and drinking
e. Testicular sperm aspiration + in vitro fertilization + intracytoplasmic sperm injection

4. You are in clinic, and you are seeing a 25-year-old patient who has had only one period in the last 1 year. She has no past medical history and is fit and well. What is the single most important test that you will ask for?
a. Day 2–5 FSH
b. Day 2–5 LH
c. Oestradiol
d. Random FSH
e. Random LH

5. A 28-year-old patient has come to see you in clinic because since she stopped the combined oral contraceptive pill 20 months ago, she has not had a period. She was on the pill since she was 18 but stopped it in order to conceive. She has no medical conditions and her BMI is 35. What is the correct investigation?
a. Diagnostic laparoscopy + dye test
b. Hormone profile: sex hormone-binding globulin (SHBG), free testosterone and FSH and LH and prolactin
c. HyCoSy
d. Pelvic ultrasound scan
e. MRI of pelvis to exclude pelvic mass

6. You are in the infertility clinic and the next patient is known to have polycystic ovarian syndrome (PCOS). She has been trying to conceive for the last 3 years but is finding it difficult, particularly because of her irregular menstrual cycles. She has a BMI of 29 and is on metformin, which is helping to keep her BMI less than 30. What is the correct treatment?
a. IUI
b. IVF
c. Laparoscopic ovarian drilling
d. Ovulation induction with clomifene for 6 months
e. Weight loss and review patient again in 6 months

7. Which of the following does spermatogenesis involve?
a. Condensation of the cytoplasm
b. Condensation of the nucleus
c. Formation of the acrosome
d. Formation of the neck, middle piece and tail
e. Shedding of the cytoplasm

8. Regarding the paramesonephric duct, which of the following is true?
   a. Caudally, opens into the abdominal cavity
   b. Caudally, it runs medial to the mesonephric duct after it crosses it
   c. Caudally, it runs medial to the mesonephric duct after crossing it ventrally
   d. Caudally, it runs laterally to the mesonephric duct after crossing it
   e. In midline, it fuses with the opposite mesonephric duct

9. A 28-year-old woman, known to have PCOS, has been trying to conceive for the last 3 years. She has a BMI of 23 and has failed to ovulate with six cycles of clomifene. What is next correct treatment?
   a. Advise weight loss
   b. Another cycle of clomifene citrate with metformin
   c. Laparoscopic ovarian drilling
   d. Oral combined contraception with cyproterone
   e. Start on metformin

10. Which of the following is incorrectly matched with regard to development of external genitalia in females?
    a. Genital swelling – mons pubis
    b. Genital folds – labia minora
    c. Genital swellings – labia majora
    d. Urogenital grove – vestibule
    e. Genital swellings – clitoris

11. You are in the infertility clinic, and you are seeing a short statured woman who complains of secondary amenorrhoea for the last 2 years. She is trying for a baby and she had a miscarriage 3 years ago. She has a BMI of 35 and is on amlodipine for hypertension. She asks you what you think the diagnosis is. Which of the following is correct?
    a. Androgen insensitivity syndrome
    b. Endometriosis
    c. Klinefelter's syndrome
    d. Premature ovarian failure
    e. Turner syndrome

12. The development of which of the following is not promoted by testosterone?
    a. Bulk of muscles
    b. Epididymis
    c. Seminiferous tubule
    d. Seminal vesicles
    e. Vas deferens

13. With respect to testosterone hormone in females, which of the following is false?
    a. Testosterone is predominantly bound to albumin
    b. Testosterone is predominantly bound to SHBG
    c. Testosterone bound to SHBG is biologically inactive

d. Testosterone bound to albumin is biologically active

e. Testosterone is ten times lower in females than in males

14. With regard to oestrogens, which of the following is incorrect?
    a. Estriol is bound to SHBG
    b. Oestrogen increases the hepatic synthesis of binding proteins
    c. Oestrogen stimulates endometrial growth
    d. Oestrogen reduces bowel motility
    e. Oestrogens inhibit conversion of tryptophan to serotonin

15. You are in the fertility clinic and you are seeing a 30-year-old woman with 3 years of infertility. Her cycles are irregular, and her 21-day progesterone is 10. Her BMI is 40, and her ultrasound and tubal investigations are all normal. Her husband's semen is normal. What is the correct management?
    a. Clomifene
    b. Gonadotropins
    c. Laparoscopic ovarian drilling
    d. Metformin
    e. Weight reduction advice

ANSWERS

1. c.   15%

Fifteen percent or one in six couples will be subfertile. Usually couples are offered investigations after trying to conceive for 1 year, but occasionally the investigations maybe offered earlier. For couples who are unable to have regular intercourse or for same sex couples, subfertility is defined as failure to conceive after six cycles of intrauterine insemination (IUI).

Further reading

- RCOG online learning resource. StratOG: Subfertility. https://elearning. rcog.org.uk/emqs-part-2-mrcog-online-resource-new-version/ gynaecology/subfertility

2. d.   Oligoasthenoteratozoospermia

According to World Health Organisation (WHO 2010), the normal reference range for semen analysis is as follows:
- Volume: $\geq$1.5 mL
- Total sperm count: $\geq$39 million
- Sperm concentration: $\geq$15 million/mL
- pH: $\geq$7.2
- Overall motility: $\geq$40%
- Progressive motility: $\geq$32%
- Normal forms: $\geq$4%
- Vitality: $\geq$58%

As the patient has a low sperm count, this is oligozoospermia (17 million). Since there is reduced motility (10%), this is asthenozoospermia. The reduced normal forms (3%) and reduced vitality (25%) is teratozoospermia; therefore, this is oligoasthenoteratozoospermia.

Further reading

- World Health Organisation (WHO): Sexual and reproductive health: Infertility definitions and terminology. https://www.who.int/ reproductivehealth/topics/infertility/definitions/en/
- RCOG online learning resource. StratOG: Subfertility. https://elearning. rcog.org.uk/emqs-part-2-mrcog-online-resource-new-version/ gynaecology/subfertility

3. a.   Donor insemination

The raised FSH and LH and low serum testosterone suggest primary testicular failure that is most likely secondary to the mumps orchitis. Although stopping smoking and drinking is good, it will not reverse the azoospermia.

Further reading

- NICE. Fertility problems (CG156): Assessment and treatment. September 2017. https://www.nice.org.uk/guidance/CG156

4. d.   Random FSH

FSH is the most important as it will enable us to differentiate between ovarian failure and ovarian dysfunction such as PCOS and hypogonadotropic hypogonadism. As she does not have periods, this cannot be done between days 2 and 5 and therefore has to be done randomly. LH is not as useful as FSH, and oestradiol cannot different between hypogonadotropic hypogonadism and ovarian dysfunction as in both the oestradiol will be low.

Further reading

- NICE. Fertility problems (CG156): Assessment and treatment. September 2017. https://www.nice.org.uk/guidance/CG156

5. b.   Hormone profile: Sex hormone-binding globulin (SHBG), free testosterone and FSH and LH and prolactin

This patient is most likely to have PCOS, and this can be confirmed with a hormone profile. The advice at this stage is weight loss and initiating metformin.

Further reading

- NICE. Fertility problems (CG156): Assessment and treatment. September 2017. https://www.nice.org.uk/guidance/CG156

6. d.   Ovulation induction with clomifene for 6 months

The patient should be encouraged to continue to lose weight and be given ovulation induction with clomifene for 6 months.

Further reading

- NICE. Fertility problems (CG156): Assessment and treatment. September 2017. https://www.nice.org.uk/guidance/CG156

7. a.   Condensation of the cytoplasm

The changes that take place in the transformation of spermatids into spermatozoa are called spermatogenesis.

Spermatogenesis is regulated by the hormone LH. This binds to receptors in the Leydig cells and promotes testosterone production, which in turn binds to Sertoli cells to promote spermatogenesis. Sertoli cells stimulate secretion of intracellular androgen receptor proteins.

The time required for a spermatogonium to develop into a mature spermatozoon is around 64 days. Spermatozoa enter the lumen of seminiferous tubules once fully formed. Thereafter, they are pushed towards the epididymis and obtain full motility in the epididymis.

Further reading

- RCOG: StratOG: Spermatogenesis: https://elearning.rcog.org.uk/male-factor-infertility/spermatogenesis

8. c. Caudally, it runs medial to the mesonephric duct after crossing it ventrally.
    There are two mesonephric ducts (Wolffian duct system) and two paramesonephric ducts (Müllerian duct system) in the body during embryonic development of the reproductive organs. The paramesonephric duct arises from the invagination of the epithelium covering the urogenital ridge on the anterolateral surface. It opens cranially into the abdominal cavity. Caudally, it lies lateral to the mesonephric duct before crossing it ventrally. It then lies medial to the mesonephric duct. Further to this, it joins the opposite paramesonephric duct in the midline and forms the uterine cavity. In females, the paramesonephric duct gives rise to the uterus, fallopian tubes, cervix, upper third of the vagina (lower two-thirds of the vagina develop from urogenital sinus) and a vestigial or rudimentary structure called Morgagni hydatid. In males, it forms the vestigial structure called the appendix of testis.

    Further reading

    - https://en.wikipedia.org/wiki/Mesonephric_duct
    - https://en.wikipedia.org/wiki/Paramesonephric_duct

9. c. Laparoscopic ovarian drilling
    The ovarian drilling will reduce the excessive ovarian stroma in women with PCOS. This in turn will reduce the amount of ovarian androgen that is produced and hence reduction in LH, which will therefore allow ovulation to occur.

    Further reading

    - NICE. Fertility problems (CG156): Assessment and treatment. September 2017. https://www.nice.org.uk/guidance/CG156

10. d. Genital swellings – clitoris
    The clitoris arises from the genital tubercle.

    Further reading

    - RCOG online source: Embryology: https://elearning.rcog.org.uk/ benign-vulval-problems/anatomy/embryology

11. e. Turner syndrome
    Patients with Turner syndrome tend to be short, obese and suffer from hypertension. They have gonadal dysgenesis and have a limited period of ovulation which enables them to get pregnant. The diagnosis is made by karyotyping, and the only treatment is egg donation.

    Further reading

    - RCOG online learning resource. StratOG: Subfertility. https://elearning. rcog.org.uk/emqs-part-2-mrcog-online-resource-new-version/ gynaecology/subfertility

12. c. Seminiferous tubule

Luteinizing hormone regulates spermatogenesis. It binds to the receptors on Leydig cells and stimulates production of testosterone, which in turn promotes spermatogenesis by binding to Sertoli cells.

Further reading

- RCOG: StratOG: Spermatogenesis: https://elearning.rcog.org.uk/ male-factor-infertility/spermatogenesis

13. a. Testosterone is predominantly bound to albumin

Eighty-five percent of testosterone is bound to SHBG and is metabolically inactive; 10%–15% is bound to albumin and 1%–2% is free. Free and albumin-bound testosterones are biologically active.

Further reading

- RCOG online learning resource. StratOG: Subfertility. https://elearning. rcog.org.uk/emqs-part-2-mrcog-online-resource-new-version/ gynaecology/subfertility

14. a. Estriol is bound to SHBG

Estriol is not bound to SHBG. Both oestrogens and progesterones are produced by the ovary. Oestrogen stimulates endometrial growth and uterine growth. Both oestrogen and progesterone reduce bowel motility. Progesterone increases the respiratory drive and the body temperature and promotes sodium secretion.

Further reading

- RCOG online learning resource. StratOG: Subfertility. https://elearning. rcog.org.uk/emqs-part-2-mrcog-online-resource-new-version/ gynaecology/subfertility

15. e. Weight reduction advice

Weight reduction to a BMI of at least less than 30 itself can help increase the chances of conceiving.

Further reading

- NICE. Fertility problems (CG156): Assessment and treatment. September 2017. https://www.nice.org.uk/guidance/CG156

KNOWLEDGE AREA 12: SEXUAL AND REPRODUCTIVE HEALTH

QUESTIONS

1. Which of the following regarding the combined oral contraceptive pills (COCP) is true?
   a. Increase the levels of antithrombin III
   b. Increase the levels of FSH by stimulating its secretion
   c. Decrease the levels of LH by inhibiting its secretion
   d. Decrease the levels of iron
   e. Increase the levels of copper

2. Regarding herpes simplex virus (HSV), which of the following statements is incorrect?
   a. Type 1 HSV is spread by direct contact
   b. Type 1 HSV is spread by droplet infection
   c. Type 1 HSV affects the genital area and oral area
   d. Type 1 HSV can cause painful gingivostomatitis
   e. Type 1 HSV can cause ocular lesions

3. A 25-year-old patient comes to see you in clinic. She is complaining of post-coital bleeding, a sore throat and a painful left knee. What is the most likely diagnosis?
   a. Bacterial vaginosis (BV)
   b. *Chlamydia trachomatis*
   c. Molluscum contagiosum
   d. Neisseria *gonorrhoeae*
   e. *Trichomonas vaginalis*

4. A 20-year-old university student comes to see you in accident and emergency (A&E) department because she has an offensive, yellowish-green frothy vaginal discharge, itching of the genital area, dysuria and dyspareunia. The discharge is causing her much anguish, she is extremely embarrassed by it and it is affecting her sex life.
   What is the most likely diagnosis?
   a. BV
   b. *C. trachomatis*

    c.   Molluscum contagiosum

    d.   *N. gonorrhoeae*

    e.   *T. vaginalis*

5. You are asked to see a 25-year-old woman who has presented with small warty lumps on the vulva skin. On examination you find multiple, small (<0.5 cm) solid lesions with umbilication in the centre (central depression). She says that her boyfriend has the same things on his body. What is the treatment?

    a.   Azithromycin

    b.   Cefuroxime

    c.   Co-amoxiclave

    d.   Conservative management

    e.   Metronidazole

6. You are the gynaecology senior house officer (SHO) on call, and the general practitioner (GP) calls you for advice. He is seeing a 21-year-old patient who has recently become sexually active. She is complaining of a grey vaginal discharge with a fishy odour. It is particularly worse after sex. What treatment would you advise?

    a.   Azithromycin

    b.   Cefuroxime

    c.   Co-amoxiclave

    d.   Conservative management

    e.   Metronidazole

7. Regarding *C. trachomatis*, which of the following statements is incorrect?

    a.   Is a facultative intracellular bacterium

    b.   Is causative organism for lymphogranuloma venereum

    c.   Is the commonest cause of non-gonococcal urethritis in men

    d.   Is the most common cause of PID in women

    e.   Can cause pneumonia in neonate

8. You are the gynaecology SHO, and you have been called by a GP for some advice. He is seeing a 34-year-old woman who is in para 1 in his clinic, and she is requesting emergency contraception. She had unprotected intercourse with two different men 4 days ago, and although initially she did not mind getting pregnant, she now wants to avoid pregnancy. She has no past medical history and is not on any medication. What is your advice?

    a.   Copper IUCD

    b.   ellaOne

    c.   Intrauterine system insertion

    d.   Levonelle

    e.   Norethisterone tablet

9. A 16-year-old girl comes to her GP as she would like to terminate her pregnancy. She is terminating as this is an unplanned pregnancy. She is currently 6 weeks pregnant. She has no past medical history of note and is not on any medications. Under which clause does this termination come under?
   a. A
   b. B
   c. C
   d. D
   e. E

10. A 15-year-old girl comes to see her GP, requesting a termination of pregnancy. What is the most important aspect of the consultation?
   a. Assessing to see if she is Fraser competent
   b. Checking her haemoglobin level, in case she needs a blood transfusion
   c. Checking her rhesus status in case she is resus negative
   d. Making sure her legal guardian is informed
   e. Making sure her boy friend is informed

11. Combined oral contraceptive pills (COCP) do not increase the risk of which of the following conditions?
   a. Deep venous thrombosis
   b. Haemorrhagic strokes in women with hypertension
   c. Hepatocellular adenoma
   d. Ischaemic stroke in women with migraine
   e. Trophoblastic disease

12. Which of the following is true regarding starting time of combined oral contraceptive pill?
   a. First day of menstruation
   b. Tenth day after delivery (non-lactating woman)
   c. 1 month after molar pregnancy
   d. Seventh day after induced early abortion
   e. Tenth day after induced late abortion

ANSWERS

1. c. Decrease the blood levels of LH by inhibiting its secretion

   COCP inhibits pituitary secretion of FSH and LH secretion and thereby inhibits follicular development in ovaries. This causes inhibition of ovulation, which is primary action of COCP.

   Further reading

   - FSRH clinical guideline: Combined hormonal contraception (January 2019, Amended July 2019. https://www.fsrh.org/ standards-and-guidance/documents/combined-hormonal-contraception/

2. b. Type 1 HSV is spread by droplet infection

   HSV is a DNA virus. HSVs are of two types (type 1 and type 2). Type 1 HSV usually causes cold sores (which can be recurrent as the virus remains latent in dorsal root ganglia and trigeminal ganglia) and ocular lesions and can also cause genital lesions in 50% of cases (orogenital contact). The cell-mediated immunity develops after the infection. It can cause recurrent attacks in individuals with immunosuppression and HIV. It can auto-innoculate into areas of trauma and present as painful blisters (herpetic whitlow).

   Type 2 usually causes genital lesions. It is sexually transmitted and often symptomatic, and it causes painful vesicles in the genital area (primary genital herpes) with fever, myalgia and autonomic neuropathy (causing bladder atony and retention of urine). This may need catheterization and hospitalization. The incubation period is 3 weeks. Anti-HSV antibodies form after an attack and recurrent attacks could be less severe, of shorter duration with fewer constitutional symptoms and less viral shedding in the presence of anti-HSV antibodies. Asymptomatic shedding of the virus can also occur.

   It can cause other complications, including corneal ulceration, erythema multiforme and eczema herpeticum.

   During pregnancy, HSV may cause fetal infection in the perinatal period. Most infections in neonates occur if the infection in the mother is a primary, that is first time, genital HSV infection and is transmitted to the fetus during its travel through the birth canal. The risk of transmission to the fetus or neonate is much lower (around 3%) with recurrent herpes due to transfer of passive immunity.

   Caesarean section is recommended in women if the primary attack of genital HSV infection is within 6 weeks of labour or lesions are visible at the time of labour (there is no benefit of caesarean section if the membranes have ruptured for more than 4 hours). Paediatricians need to be informed as it can cause serious infections in the neonate, including disseminated disease (mortality rate = 70%–80%). It can cause life-threatening pneumonia and encephalitis (mortality rate >90%) in the newborn with long-term sequelae.

   The Tzanck test is used to demonstrate multinucleate giant cells. Also swabs from vesicle fluid can be taken for culture. Treatment of genital lesions is mainly supportive (pain relief and treatment of secondary infection). Oral aciclovir (200 mg five times a day for 5 days) is used in cases of primary genital HSV, and this may shorten the duration of symptoms.

Further reading

- RCOG guideline (Joint guideline with BASSH). Management of genital herpes in pregnancy. October 2014. https://www.rcog.org.uk/en/guidelines-research-services/guidelines/genital-herpes/
- British Association of Sexual Health and HIV (BASHH) guidelines: https://bashh.org/guidelines
- https://www.bing.com/search?q=herpesbashh+guidelines&qs=n&form=QBRE&sp=-1&pq=herpebashh+guidelines&sc=1-21&sk=&cvid=08EDFDBDF71D41FFB0A9BDFEF8C474EB

3. d.   *Neisseria gonorrhoeae*

N. gonorrhoeae is a Gram-negative diplococcus. This organism can be seen within the cytoplasm of polymorphs on Gram staining. It can cause urethritis (males) and cervicitis (females), proctitis, pharyngitis and septic arthritis. It can also cause conjunctivitis in the newborn acquired during its passage through the birth canal.

Further reading

- BASHH guidelines: https://bashh.org/guidelines
- https://www.bing.com/search?q=N.+gonorrhoeae++bashh+guidelines&qs=n&form=QBRE&sp=-1&pq=n.+gonorrhoeae+bashh+guidelines&sc=0-31&sk=&cvid=0302052ACEA74661BF1758B5D20004B5

4. e.   *T. vaginalis*

T. vaginalis (TV) is a single-celled, flagellated, motile protozoan. It is slightly larger than a granulocyte and depends on adherence to the host cell for its survival. Women can present with yellowish-green frothy vaginal discharge (has odour), itching of the genital area, dysuria and dyspareunia (vaginitis, cervicitis and urethritis). It may lead to premature rupture of membranes and preterm delivery. It can coexist with other genital infections such as gonorrhoea, *Chlamydia* and BV. Most men are usually asymptomatic and can (rarely) develop genital irritation, epididymitis and prostatitis.

On speculum examination, the vaginal mucosa is erythematous and the cervix is inflamed with numerous petechiae (strawberry appearance). Motile organisms are seen on wet mount saline preparation under the microscope.

Wet mount microscopy and culture are the gold standard for its diagnosis. Metronidazole is the drug of choice for this treatment.

Further reading

- BASHH guidelines: https://bashh.org/guidelines
- https://www.bing.com/search?q=tricomonas+vaginalis+bashh+guidelines&qs=n&form=QBRE&sp=-1&pq=tricomonas+vagi+bashh+guidelines&sc=0-32&sk=&cvid=CC06DF596D4E451E8FC0B154A7467749

5. d. Conservative management

This patient has molluscum contagiosum, which is a common skin infection of childhood. It presents as multiple, small, umbilicated (the lesions have a central depression called a punctum), solid lesions on skin (<0.5 cm) and can occur anywhere in the body. Occasionally, they can reach 1 cm in size and are called giant molluscum. The spread is by direct contact, and scratching promotes its spread. As they resolve spontaneously, they rarely require treatment.

Further reading

● BASHH guidelines: https://bashh.org/guidelines
● https://www.bing.com/search?q=molluscum+contagiosum+bashh+gu idelines&qs=n&form=QBRE&sp=-1&pq=molluscum+contagiosum+b ashh+guidelines&sc=1-38&sk=&cvid=603A348488EB4DDAA0ECE80 015EDFD52

6. e. Metronidazole

This patient has bacterial vaginosis (BV), a polymicrobial superficial vaginal infection due to an overgrowth of anaerobes and is the most common cause of vaginal discharge. *Gardnerella vaginalis* (also known as *Haemophilus vaginalis*) is a facultative, anaerobic, non-flagellated, non-spore-forming bacterium. It is recognized as one of the organisms responsible for causing BV. The other organisms involved in this pathology are *Bacteroides, Peptostreptococcus, Fusobacterium, Mycoplasma hominis, Mobiluncus* and *Veilonella*.

Women present with thin grey homogeneous vaginal discharge and a characteristic fishy odour (alkalinity of semen may cause a release of volatile amines from the vaginal discharge – forms the basis for the whiff test). The fishy smell is mainly recognized after sexual intercourse. Vulval itching, dysuria and dyspareunia are rare. It is also known to cause vault infection following hysterectomy and pelvic infection after abortion. In pregnant women, it has been associated with premature rupture of membranes and preterm delivery. The following are recognized as risk factors for the development of BV: vaginal douching, antibiotic use, decrease in oestrogen production, presence of intrauterine device and increase in number of sexual partners.

There is an increase in vaginal pH as it is associated with a decrease in lactobacilli (responsible for maintaining the acidic pH) in the vagina. Wet mount saline preparation with vaginal discharge shows clue cells (vaginal epithelial cells have a stippled appearance due to adherence of coccobacilli) under low- and high-power microscopy. The drug used for treatment is metronidazole (single dose of 2 g or 7-day course of oral dose [500 mg bd for 7 days]). Metronidazole is contraindicated during early pregnancy. Topical clindamycin and metronidazole are also useful in returning the vaginal flora to normal.

Amsel's criteria for diagnosis of BV are (a) thin white homogeneous discharge; (b) increase in vaginal pH (4.5); (c) clue cells on microscopy and (d) whiff test – when a few drops of alkali (10% KOH) are added to vaginal secretions, a fishy smell is released. At least three of the four criteria should be present to make the diagnosis.

Further reading

- BASHH guidelines: https://bashh.org/guidelines
- https://www.bing.com/search?q=bacterial+vaginosis+bashh+guidelines&FORM=AWRE

7. a. Is a facultative intracellular bacterium

C. trachomatis is an obligate intracellular pathogen and cannot grow outside a living cell. *Chlamydia* infection is a sexually transmitted infection. Certain strains of *C. trachomatis* (serovars A, B, Ba, C) are associated with trachoma, which is a major cause of blindness worldwide. Serovars L1, L2 and L3 are associated with lymphogranuloma venereum. Serovars D to K cause non-specific urethritis and epididymitis in men and perihepatitis, cervicitis, urethritis, endometritis and salpingitis (infection of upper genital tract – leading to PID) in women. It can cause Reiter syndrome in both men and women (conjunctivitis, proctitis, urethritis and reactive seronegative arthritis). Its long-term sequelae include chronic pelvic pain, infertility and ectopic pregnancy. It is associated with increased rates of transmission of HIV infection. It can be transmitted to the neonate during its passage through the birth canal and may cause conjunctivitis and pneumonia.

The incubation period is 1–3 weeks and men present with mucopurulent urethral discharge (urethritis) and women present with vaginal discharge (cervicitis). Asymptomatic infection is not uncommon in both men and women. Cervical or urethral swabs (first sample of urine in men) are collected for culture and nucleic acid amplification test. It is sensitive to doxycycline and erythromycin group of drugs.

Further reading

- BASHH guidelines: https://bashh.org/guidelines
- https://www.bing.com/search?q=bash+guidelines+chlamydia&FORM=R5FD2

8. a. Copper IUCD

ellaOne is a selective progesterone receptor modulator. It can be used up to 120 hours after unprotected intercourse. Levonelle is levonorgesterol 1500 mg, and it can be used up to 72 hours after intercourse. The copper IUCD is the most effective of the emergency contraception and can be inserted up to 120 hours after intercourse. The intrauterine system and norethisterone are not licenced as an emergency contraceptive.

Further reading

- Faculty of Sexual and Reproductive Healthcare (FSRH). https://www.fsrh.org/standards-and-guidance/documents/ceuguidanceintrauterinecontraception/
- Intrauterine contraception: Faculty of Sexual and Reproductive Healthcare. June 2015. https://www.guidelines.co.uk/womens-health/fsrh-intrauterine-contraception-guideline/252622.article

9. c.   C

The clauses of termination of pregnancy are categorized as follows:

A	The continuance of the pregnancy would involve risk to the life of the pregnant woman greater than if the pregnancy were terminated
B	The termination is necessary to prevent grave permanent injury to the physical or mental health of the pregnant woman
C	The continuance of the pregnancy would involve risk, greater than if the pregnancy were terminated, of injury to the physical or mental health of the pregnant woman
D	The continuance of the pregnancy would involve risk, greater than if the pregnancy were terminated, of injury to the physical or mental health of any existing children in the family of the pregnant woman
E	There is a substantial risk that if the child were born, it would suffer from such physical or mental abnormalities as to be seriously handicapped, or in an emergency, certified by the operating practitioner as immediately necessary: • (F) to save the life of the pregnant woman • (G) to prevent grave permanent injury to the physical or mental health of the pregnant woman

In the United Kingdom, 98% of clauses are carried out under clause C.

Further Reading

- RCOG online learning resource. StratOG: Fertility control and contraception. https://elearning.rcog.org.uk/fertility-control-and-contraception/fertility-control-and-contraception

10. a.   Assessing to see if she is Fraser competent

In England and Wales, a patient under the age of 16 is able to give consent to a termination if she is Fraser competent. This means that she is able to understand the information given to her. The decision as to whether the patient is Fraser competent is at the discretion of the doctor.

Further reading

- UNDER-16S: Consent and confidentiality in sexual health services. https://www.fpa.org.uk/factsheets/under-16s-consent-and-confidentiality-sexual-health-services

- RCOG online learning resource. StratOG: Fertility
  control and contraception. https://elearning.rcog.org.uk/
  fertility-control-and-contraception/fertility-control-and-contraception

11. a. Deep venous thrombosis

   COCPs increase the risk of thromboembolism (deep venous thrombosis
   and pulmonary embolism), myocardial infarction and thrombotic strokes.
   It shows no association with prolactinomas and trophoblastic disease.

   Further reading

   - FSRH clinical guideline: Combined hormonal contraception. January 2019,
     Amended July 2019. https://www.fsrh.org/standards-and-guidance/
     documents/combined-hormonal-contraception/

12. a. First day of menstruation

   In lactating women, COCP is started on day 21 post-delivery. Post-
   abortion, COCP is usually started same day or next day.

   Further reading

   - FSRH clinical guideline: Combined hormonal contraception. January 2019,
     Amended July 2019. https://www.fsrh.org/standards-and-guidance/
     documents/combined-hormonal-contraception/

KNOWLEDGE AREA 13: EARLY PREGNANCY CARE

QUESTIONS

1. Which of the following hormones is not produced by the corpus luteum?
   a. Inhibin A
   b. Inhibin B
   c. Activin
   d. Relaxin
   e. Progesterone

2. You (speciality trainee year 2) are working in the early pregnancy unit and the sonographer asks you to review a patient. Two sonographers have performed a scan on a patient and are unsure regarding what to advise the patient. She is 34-year-old primigravida who is 6 weeks pregnant by date. Her periods are irregular, and she is very worried as she has been spotting. The report reads as follows:

   > Transvaginal scan performed with chaperone and consent. Intrauterine gestation sac 25 mm and fetal pole seen with crown rump length of 6 mm but with no fetal heartbeat. Right ovary 23 × 33 × 43 mm and contains the corpus luteum. Left ovary measures 43 × 50 × 20 mm and contains simple cyst of 3 cm. No adnexal masses, adnexal tenderness or free fluid. Patient was advised to see the doctor.

   What is your management plan?
   a. Offer condolences and advise surgical management
   b. Offer condolences and advise conservative management
   c. Offer condolences and advise medical management
   d. Rescan in 7–10 days
   e. Seek a third opinion

3. You (senior house officer or speciality trainee year 2) are working in the early pregnancy unit and the sonographer asks you to review a patient. Two sonographers have performed a scan on a patient and are unsure regarding what to advise the patient. She is a 34-year-old primigravida who is 6 weeks pregnant by date. Her periods have always been irregular and she is worried as she has been having vaginal red spotting. The scan report reads as follows:

Transvaginal scan performed with chaperone and consent. Intrauterine gestation sac 25 mm and fetal pole seen with crown rump length of 10 mm but with no fetal heartbeat. Right ovary 23 × 33 × 43 mm. Left ovary measures 43 × 50 × 20 mm and contains the corpus luteum. No adnexal masses, adnexal tenderness or free fluid. Patient was advised to see doctor.

What is your management plan?
a. Offer condolences and advise surgical management
b. Offer condolences and advise conservative management
c. Offer condolences and advise medical management
d. Rescan in 7–10 days
e. Seek a third opinion

4. You (senior house officer or speciality trainee year 2) are on call, and you receive a call from accident and emergency (A&E) department to examine a patient who is 6 weeks pregnant and is having vaginal bleeding. Upon arrival you find the patient has crampy abdominal pain and has soaked eight pads. On examination you find that her abdomen is soft and there is no guarding or rebound tenderness. Her BP is 80/40 mmHg and her pulse 112 beats per minute despite having 2 L of Hartman's solution, intravenous fluid through an intravenous cannula. Her temperature is 36.8°. She is unable to pass urine to give a sample for a pregnancy test. She said she has had an ultrasound scan 2 days ago and the report is as follows:

Transvaginal scan performed with chaperone and consent. Intrauterine gestation sac and fetal pole seen with crown rump length of 6 mm but with no fetal heartbeat. Right ovary 23 × 33 × 43 mm and contains the corpus luteum. Left ovary measures 43 × 50 × 20 mm. No adnexal masses, adnexal tenderness or free fluid. Patient advised to see the doctor.

What is your management plan?
a. Offer condolences and advise surgical management
b. Offer condolences and advise conservative management
c. Offer condolences and advise medical management
d. Rescan in 7–10 days
e. Seek a third opinion

5. You (senior house officer or speciality trainee year 2) are working in the early pregnancy unit, and the sonographer asks you to review a patient. Two sonographers have performed a scan on a patient and are unsure regarding what to advise the patient. She is a 34-year-old primigravida who is 6 weeks pregnant by date and has regular periods. She is very worried as she has been having vaginal spotting. The report reads as follows:

Transvaginal scan performed with chaperone and consent. No intrauterine pregnancy seen. Right ovary 23 × 33 × 43 mm. Adjacent to the right ovary was seen a mass moving separately to the right ovary measuring 24 × 21 × 20 mm, suggestive most likely tubal ectopic pregnancy. Left ovary measures 43 × 50 × 20 mm. No adnexal tenderness or free fluid. Patient was advised to see doctor.

A BHCG was performed and the levels were 166 IU/L.
What is your management plan?

a. Abdominal salpingectomy
b. Conservative management
c. Laparoscopic salpingectomy
d. Methotrexate
e. Repeat serum hCG in 48 hours

6. You (senior house officer or speciality trainee year 2) are working in the early pregnancy unit and the sonographer asks you to review a patient. She is a 34-year-old primigravida who is 6 weeks pregnant by date and has irregular periods. She is very worried as she has been having abdominal pain and mild vaginal spotting. Two sonographers have performed a scan on the patient and are unsure regarding what to advise. The report reads as follows:

> Transvaginal scan performed with chaperone and consent. No intrauterine pregnancy seen. Right ovary 23 × 33 × 43 mm. Adjacent to the right ovary was seen a mass moving separately to the right ovary measuring 23 × 24 × 30 mm. Left ovary measures 43 × 50 × 20 mm. No adnexal tenderness or free fluid. Patient was advised to see the doctor.

A serum hCG was performed and the levels were 6324 IU/L.
What is your management plan?

a. Abdominal salpingectomy
b. Conservative management
c. Laparoscopic salpingectomy
d. Methotrexate
e. Repeat serum hCG in 48 hours

7. A 40-year-old woman underwent a surgical management of miscarriage for a missed miscarriage. The histopathology has returned as molar pregnancy. She is very upset with the diagnosis as she has heard that this is not a normal pregnancy and not a common condition.

   She asks you what is the incidence of this condition. Which of the following options is correct?

a. 1:500–1:1000 pregnancies
b. 1:1000–1:2000 pregnancies
c. 1:2000–1:3000 pregnancies
d. 1:3000–1:4000 pregnancies
e. 1:4000–1:5000 pregnancies

8. A 40-year-old woman underwent a surgical management of miscarriage for a missed miscarriage 10 weeks ago. The histopathology had returned as molar pregnancy. She had a serum BCG at the hospital 24 hours ago and the levels were 1150 IU/L.

   How long should she be followed up for?

a. 3 months from when she had the uterine evacuation
b. 3 months from the date the serum HCG is normalized
c. 3 months from when the histology results returned

    d. 6 months from when she had the uterine evacuation

    e. 6 months from the date the serum HCG is normalized

9. You (senior house officer or speciality trainee year 2) are on call and the local general practitioner (GP) gives you a telephone call to ask advice for a patient. She is a 35-year-old patient who was diagnosed with a molar pregnancy, following a surgical evacuation of retained products and is still being followed up as her serum HCG has not normalized yet. She wants contraception now.

    What is your advice?

    a. Barrier methods

    b. Combined oral contraceptive

    c. Depo injection

    d. Intrauterine device

    e. Progesterone-only contraceptive

10. When breaking bad news to a woman who has a miscarriage, which of the following is true?

    a. All women will be upset by the news of having a miscarriage

    b. Having a detached professional attitude will make the news less upsetting for the patient

    c. Having a chaperone when breaking the bad news is essential

    d. Most women will view the miscarriage as loss of a baby, regardless of gestation

    e. The earlier the gestation of the pregnancy, the less upset the patient will be

ANSWERS

1. c.   Activin

   The corpus luteum produces all the above-mentioned hormones plus oestrogen except activin.

   Further reading

   - Chard T and Lilford R. *Basic Sciences for Obstetrics and Gynaecology* (5th ed). ISBN-13: 978-3540761884.

2. d.   Rescan in 7–10 days

   If the crown rump length is less than 7 mm and there is no fetal heart beat, then the patient should have a rescan after 7 days after the first scan before making a diagnosis of miscarriage.

   Further reading

   - National Institute of Health and Care Excellence (NICE). CG154: Ectopic pregnancy and miscarriage: Diagnosis and initial management. December 2012.

3. b.   Offer condolences and advise conservative management

   If the CRL is greater than 7 mm and there is no fetal heartbeat, then a second opinion should be sought and/or a second scan performed in 7 days. In this scenario, the second opinion has already been sought and therefore the diagnosis is miscarriage. The initial management should be conservative.

   Further reading

   - National Institute of Health and Care Excellence (NICE). Ectopic pregnancy and miscarriage: Diagnosis and initial management. CG154. December 2012.

4. a.   Offer condolences and advise surgical management

   This patient is haemodynamically compromised; explain the situation to the patient and advise surgical management as soon as possible.

   Further reading

   - National Institute of Health and Care Excellence (NICE). Ectopic pregnancy and miscarriage: Diagnosis and initial management. CG154. December 2012.

5. d.   Methotrexate

   Methotrexate should be advised as first-line treatment in the following women:
   - If they can return for follow-up
   - No intrauterine pregnancy
   - No significant pain

- Unruptured ectopic
- Mass less than 35 mm and no visible heartbeat
- Serum hCG less than 1500 IU/L

Further reading

- National Institute of Health and Care Excellence (NICE). Ectopic pregnancy and miscarriage: Diagnosis and initial management. CG154. December 2012.
- Royal College of Obstetricians and Gynaecologists (RCOG). Diagnosis and management of ectopic pregnancy. November 2016.

6. c.   Laparoscopic salpingectomy
Surgery should be advised if any of the following are present:

- Significant pain
- The adnexal mass is 35 mm or more
- The ectopic pregnancy has a fetal heartbeat
- The serum hCG is greater than 5000 IU/L

As this patient is stable, so the laparoscopic approach can be taken.

Further reading

- National Institute of Health and Care Excellence (NICE). Ectopic pregnancy and miscarriage: Diagnosis and initial management. CG154. December 2012.
- Royal College of Obstetricians and Gynaecologists (RCOG). Diagnosis and management of ectopic pregnancy. November 2016.

7. a.   1:500–1:1000
The incidence is 1:714 pregnancies. The incidence is higher in women of Asian ethnicity than non-Asian.

Further reading

- Royal College of Obstetricians and Gynaecologists (RCOG). The Management of Gestational Trophoblastic Disease. February 2010.
- StratOG eLearning. RCOG online resource. Gynaecological problems and early pregnancy loss. https://stratog.rcog.org.uk/tutorials/core-knowledge/gynaecological-problems-and-early-pregnancy-loss/early-pregnancy-loss

8. e.   6 months from the date the serum HCG is normalized
Follow-up should be individualized.

- If the serum HCG normalizes within 56 days of the pregnancy, then the follow-up is 6 months from the date of the evacuation.
- If the serum HCG does not normalize within 56 days of the pregnancy, then the follow-up is for 6 months following the normalization of the serum HCG.

- If the patient then has a normal pregnancy, she should have a serum HCG 6-8 after giving birth to ensure there is no disease recurrence.

Further reading

- Royal College of Obstetricians and Gynaecologists (RCOG). The Management of Gestational Trophoblastic Disease. February 2010.
- StratOG eLearning. RCOG online learning resource. *Gynaecological Problems and Early Pregnancy Loss.* https://stratog.rcog.org.uk/tutorials/core-knowledge/gynaecological-problems-and-early-pregnancy-loss/early-pregnancy-loss
- StratOG eLearning. RCOG online resource. Maternal medicine - Neoplasia in pregnancy

9. a. Barrier methods

Patients who have had a molar pregnancy should use barrier methods until the serum HCG has normalized. Only once they have normalized can the combined oral contraceptive be used. However, if the combined oral contraceptive pill is already started before the diagnosis of a molar pregnancy was made, then the patient should continue the pill as it does not appear to increase the risk of gestational trophoblastic neoplasia (invasive mole or choriocarcinomas). Therefore, women can be advised to continue the oral contraceptive pills following evacuation of molar pregnancy and before the hCG has returned to normal. They should also be advised to use the pills to avoid pregnancy until the surveillance is completed.

Intrauterine contraceptive devise should not be used until the serum HCG has normalized due to the risk of perforation.

Further reading

- Royal College of Obstetricians and Gynaecologists (RCOG). The Management of Gestational Trophoblastic Disease. February 2010.
- StratOG eLearning. RCOG online resource. *Gynaecological Problems and Early Pregnancy Loss.* https://stratog.rcog.org.uk/tutorials/core-knowledge/gynaecological-problems-and-early-pregnancy-loss/early-pregnancy-loss
- Ngan HY, Seckl MJ, Berkowitz RS et al. Update on the diagnosis and management of gestational trophoblastic disease. *International Journal of Gynecology & Obstetrics.* 2015; 2(1):S123–S126. doi: 10.1016/j.ijgo.2015.06.008.

10. d. Most women will view the miscarriage as loss of a baby, regardless of gestation

Not all women will be upset by having a miscarriage, as to some it may come as a relief of an unwanted pregnancy. Being detached as a profession will not help ease the patient's suffering and may come across as unsupportive and unempathetic. Having a chaperone to break bad news is not essential. There is no correlation with gestation and how upset a patient will be. Most, if not all, women view a miscarriage as a loss of a baby, even if it was anembryonic. Therefore, an empathetic and supportive approach is required.

Further reading

- StratOG eLearning. RCOG online resource. Early pregnancy loss— Breaking bad news. https://stratog.rcog.org.uk/tutorials/core-knowledge/gynaecological-problems-and-early-pregnancy-loss/early-pregnancy-loss-0

QUESTIONS

1. A routine screening test is available to identify lesions early during precancerous stage in which of the following organs?
   a. Cervix
   b. Endometrium
   c. Fallopian tube
   d. Ovary
   e. Vulva

2. A 66-year-old woman is seen in gynaecological oncology clinic. She complains of bloating for the past 4 months. Her ca125 levels are 100 u/mL and an ultrasound scan shows bilateral multicystic ovarian masses with solid components in it.
   What is the risk of malignancy index (RMI) in her case?
   a. 180
   b. 250
   c. 300
   d. 600
   e. 900

3. A 67-year-old woman is seen in gynaecological oncology clinic in a cancer unit. She presents with 6-month history of bloating and gradual distension of abdomen. Her bowel and bladder functions are normal. Her ultrasound scan of abdomen and pelvis shows right adnexal solid ovarian mass with moderate ascites and omental thickening. Her ca125 level is 290 u/mL.
   What is your initial management in her case?
   a. Arrange MRI scan of the pelvis with contrast to characterize the mass
   b. Arrange omental biopsy
   c. Arrange ascetic tap for cytology
   d. Refer her to cancer centre
   e. Repeat ca125 blood test

4. A 28-year-old woman presents to the emergency gynaecology service with abdominal pain. Clinical examination reveals a large abdo-pelvic mass. An MRI scan of the pelvis suggests germ cell tumour. She undergoes fertility sparing surgery at a cancer centre. The histology is reported as endodermal sinus tumour of right ovary.

   Which of the following tumour markers is specific to the tumour she has been diagnosed?
   a. Alpha-fetoprotein (AFP)
   b. Ca-125
   c. Carcinoembryoic antigen
   d. Human chorionic gonadotropin
   e. Lactate dehydrogenase (LDH)

5. A 20-year-old woman is referred to a 2 week wait gynaecological oncology clinic with abdominal distention and pain. Examination reveals a pelvic mass. An ultrasound scan reveals a mixed solid and cystic mass in the right ovary. The solid component is vascular on Doppler study. A further imaging MRI scan of the pelvis and CT scan of chest/abdomen and pelvis show suspected germ cell malignancy of the right ovarian mass and normal left ovary. She undergoes staging laparotomy and fertility sparing surgery at cancer centre. The histology of the right ovarian tumour reveals Schiller–Duval bodies.

   What is the histological type of tumour in her case?
   a. Dysgerminoma
   b. Endodermal sinus tumour
   c. Embryonal carcinoma
   d. Choriocarcinoma
   e. Immature teratoma

6. A 22-year-old woman is referred to a 2 week wait gynaecological oncology clinic with abdominal distention and pain. Examination reveals a pelvic mass. An ultrasound scan reveals large mass on the right ovary. A further imaging MRI scan of the pelvis and CT scan of chest/abdomen and pelvis show a large lobulated mass with enhancing septum. A high suspicion of germ cell malignancy is suggested in the multidisciplinary meeting at the cancer centre. She undergoes staging laparotomy and fertility sparing surgery at a cancer centre. The histology of the right ovarian mass reveals nests of cells with eosinophilic cytoplasm resembling primordial cells separated by fibrous stroma infiltrated with mature T lymphocytes.

   What is the histological type of tumour in her case?
   a. Dysgerminoma
   b. Endodermal sinus tumour
   c. Embryonal carcinoma
   d. Choriocarcinoma
   e. Immature teratoma

7. A 22-year-old nulliparous woman is referred to a 2 week wait gynaecological oncology clinic with abdominal distention and pain. Examination reveals a pelvic mass. An ultrasound scan reveals a large lobulated solid mass on the right ovary. A further imaging MRI scan of the pelvis and CT scan of chest/abdomen and pelvis show a large lobulated mass with enhancing septum. Her serum LDH is increased. A high suspicion of germ cell malignancy (dysgerminomas) is indicated in the multidisciplinary meeting at cancer centre.

    The principles of management in her case include all except which of the following?
    a. Surgery at specialist cancer centre
    b. Fertility sparing surgery in young women
    c. Staging the extent of disease
    d. Biopsy of contralateral ovary
    e. Selective removal of enlarged lymph nodes

8. A 16-year-old woman presents to emergency gynaecology with abdomen distention and pain. Ultrasound scan of abdomen and pelvis shows solid/cystic mass. Her tumour markers reveal raised AFP and beta-human chorionic gonadotropin (β-hCG). A germ cell tumour is indicated on staging CT scan following discussion at multidisciplinary meeting at cancer centre.

    What is the likely diagnosis in her case?
    a. Choriocarcinoma
    b. Dysgerminoma
    c. Embryonal carcinoma
    d. Immature teratoma
    e. Yolk sac tumour

9. An 18-year-old woman presents to emergency gynaecology with abdomen distention and pain. Ultrasound scan of abdomen and pelvis shows large abdominal mass. Her tumour markers AFP, β-hCG and LDH levels are normal. A malignant germ cell tumour is indicated on staging CT scan and MRI scan of the pelvis following discussion at multidisciplinary meeting at cancer centre. She undergoes a fertility sparing surgery at a cancer centre (laparotomy, right salpingo-oophorectomy, omentectomy, washings and peritoneal biopsies). The final histology reveals immature neuroepithelial tissue, grade 1.

    What is the likely histological diagnosis in her case?
    a. Choriocarcinoma
    b. Dysgerminoma
    c. Embryonal carcinoma
    d. Immature teratoma
    e. Yolk sac tumour

10. A 36-year-old woman is referred to the gynaecology clinic with an ultrasound scan report of dermoid cyst on the right ovary measuring 15 × 14 cm. She undergoes a laparotomy and right oophorectomy. The histology of the right ovarian cyst is predominantly thyroid tissue.
    What is the likely histological diagnosis in her case?
    a. Angiosarcoma of the ovary
    b. Carcinosarcoma of the ovary
    c. Carcinoid tumour of the ovary
    d. Struma ovarii of the ovary
    e. Squamous cell carcinoma arising in dermoid cyst

11. A patient attends colposcopy following an abnormal smear result. Colposcopic examination revealed dense acetowhite area, and therefore a cervix biopsy was taken and sent for urgent histology. The result shows CIN III.
    Which of the following is the most likely cause?
    a. HPV 6
    b. HSV 2
    c. HSV 1
    d. HPV 1
    e. HPV 16

12. A patient has an abnormal smear, and biopsy results are reported as high-grade CGIN.
    This patient is at increased risk of which of the following?
    a. Endometrial carcinoma
    b. Adenocarcinoma of cervix
    c. Serous ovarian carcinoma
    d. Endometrioid endometrial carcinoma
    e. Cervical sarcoma

13. A 4-year-old girl presents to her GP with a grape-like polypoid mass protruding through her introitus. Which of the following is the most likely diagnosis?
    a. Squamous cell carcinoma
    b. Leiomyoma
    c. Adenocarcinoma
    d. Rhabdomyosarcoma
    e. Dysgerminoma

14. A woman presents with a positive urine pregnancy test and intractable nausea and vomiting with 4+ ketones on urine dip. Transvaginal ultrasound scan shows no intrauterine pregnancy but a large echogenic mass with innumerable anechoic spaces (granular appearance). The serum BHCG level is 10,524.
    What is the most likely diagnosis?
    a. Molar pregnancy
    b. Choriocarcinoma
    c. Granulosa cell tumour

   d. Endometrial carcinoma
   e. Pituitary adenoma

15. A 65-year-old nulliparous woman presents to A&E with shortness of breath
    and dry cough. She is admitted under the acute medical team. X-ray confirmed
    a right-sided pleural effusion, and clinical examination shows ascites. No
    malignant cells are identified in the pleural aspirate or ascetic fluid. There was
    a large, firm abdominal mass palpated on examination of the abdomen.
       What is the most likely explanation for this presentation?
    a. Sheehan syndrome
    b. Meigs syndrome
    c. Asherman's syndrome
    d. Neuroendocrine carcinoma
    e. Kikuchi disease

16. The risk of endometrial carcinoma is most likely to be increased by which of
    the following neoplasms?
    a. Melanoma
    b. Mesothelioma
    c. Granulosa-theca cell tumour
    d. Schwannoma
    e. Krukenberg tumour

17. A patient has had her colon removed for prophylactic reasons due to hereditary
    non-polyposis colorectal cancer.
       Which of the following is she most at risk?
    a. Cervical squamous cell carcinoma
    b. Germ cell tumours of the ovary
    c. Sex-cord tumours of the ovary
    d. Endometrial carcinoma
    e. Rhabdomyosarcoma botryoides

18. A patient is noted to have bilateral ovarian tumours, which are removed.
    The histopathology report that the tumour cells show signet ring morphology
    and raise the possibility that these represent metastasis rather than primary
    ovarian malignancy.
       Which is the most likely primary site?
    a. Cervix
    b. Uterus
    c. Pancreas
    d. Stomach
    e. Thyroid

ANSWERS

1. a.   Cervix

There are no routine screening tests for the detection of either endometrial, ovarian, fallopian tube and vulvar cancers or precancers.

Ultrasound scan of the pelvis is first and best primary modality of imaging that can be used to identify if there is any abnormality in the uterus (thickened endometrium) or to identify if there is an ovarian mass when there is a clinical suspicion. Ultrasound is also used in some women prophylactically at regular intervals when there is a family history of uterine, colon and ovarian cancer, especially when there is positive gene history in the family.

Further reading

- StratOG: RCOGs online learning resource. https://stratog.rcog. org.uk/tutorial/diagnostic-imaging-in-gynaecological-oncology/ screening-and-diagnosis-in-ovarian-cancer-5494
- RCOG: Green-top Guideline No. 24. The management of ovarian cysts in postmenopausal

2. e.   900

RMI

In case of ovarian/adnexal mass, the appearance of mass is given a score along with other features on the scan. This is further combined with ca125 blood test and menopausal status (postmenopausal woman gets a score of 3) of the woman to assess the risk of cancer, which is called risk of malignancy index (RMI). The postmenopausal status score of 3 is multiplied by the ca125 level × score of appearance of the ovarian/ adnexal mass.

The features on ultrasound scan include the following:

a. Multiloculated cysts/thick septa >3 mm
b. Bilaterality
c. Papillary projections in the cyst wall/solid components
d. Presence of ascites
e. Presence of metastasis
    Score of 0 is given for no features
    Score of 1 is given for one of the above features present
    Score of 3 is given if 2–5 of the above features are present

Further reading

- RCOG: Green-top Guideline No. 24. The management of ovarian cysts in postmenopausal women. July 2016.

3. d.   Refer her to cancer centre

If RMI is >200, the risk of ovarian cancer is high (75%), and if RMI is low (<25), then the risk of ovarian cancer is <5%. If the score is high, then these women should be referred to a cancer centre to be discussed in the multidisciplinary team meeting. If all the indicators suggest ovarian cancer, a CT scan of chest, abdomen and pelvis will be advised for staging of ovarian cancer. The woman will be offered primary debulking surgery or neoadjuvant chemotherapy depending on the CT scan findings.

The RMI in this case is 2610, which is high. The risk of ovarian cancer in her case is 75%. Therefore, the initial management is referral to the cancer centre.

Further reading

● RCOG: Green-top Guideline No. 24. The management of ovarian cysts in postmenopausal.

4. a. Alpha-fetoprotein (AFP)

The Royal College of Obstetricians and Gynecologists (RCOG) guideline recommends determination of the following tumour marker panel in women less than 40 years of age with suspected germ cell tumour of the ovary to differentiate these from epithelial ovarian cancers. These include AFP, human chorionic gonadotropin (hCG) and LDH serum levels. Only AFP and HCG are validated and studied adequately. Also, elevation of these two markers has shown to have a correlation with FIGO stage and survival in women with malignant ovarian germ cells tumours (higher levels of these markers are associated with higher FIGO stage and decreased survival and is independent of the stage).

Further reading

● Royal College of Obstetricians and Gynaecologists (RCOG). Green-top Guideline No. 62: Management of suspected ovarian masses in premenopausal women. RCOG/BSGE Joint Guideline I. November 2011. https://www.rcog.org.uk/globalassets/documents/guidelines/gtg_62.pdf
● RCOG: Scientific Impact Paper No. 52. Management of female malignant ovarian germ cell tumours. November 2016. https://www.rcog.org.uk/globalassets/documents/guidelines/scientific-impact-papers/sip_52.pdf

5. b. Endodermal sinus tumour

Schiller–Duval bodies are named after Marthias-Marie Duval and Walter Schiller. They are seen microscopically in yolk sac tumours and are present in around 50% of these tumours. Schiller–Duval body is characterized by a papilla with a fibrovascular core surrounded at the periphery by primitive epithelial cells (central vessel surrounded by tumour cells). They resemble the structure of a glomerulus and have a mesodermal core with a central capillary and are lined by flattened tumour cells. Immunofluorescent staining studies show eosinophilic hyaline-like globules both outside and inside the cytoplasm that contain alpha 1-antitrypsin and AFP. Serum AFP will be raised in women with endodermal sinus tumours.

Further reading

● Norris HJ, Jensen RD. Relative frequency of ovarian neoplasms in children and adolescents. *Cancer* 1972; 30(3):713–719.
● Royal College of Obstetricians and Gynaecologists (RCOG). Green-top Guideline No. 62: Management of suspected ovarian masses in

premenopausal women. RCOG/BSGE Joint Guideline I. November 2011. https://www.rcog.org.uk/globalassets/documents/guidelines/gtg_62.pdf

- https://en.wikipedia.org/wiki/Schiller%E2%80%93Duval_body

6. a. Dysgerminoma

Tumour infiltration with T lymphocytes is typically seen in dysgerminomas. The tumour cells are arranged in nests and separated by fibrous septa. These cells have eosinophilic cytoplasm and a central large round or flattened nucleus that contains more than one nucleoli and often have numerous mitoses.

Further reading

- Prat J. Germ cell tumors. In: Prat J, ed. *Pathology of the Ovary.* Philadelphia, PA: Saunders, 2004.
- RCOG: Scientific Impact Paper No. 52. Management of Female Malignant Ovarian Germ Cell Tumours. November 2016.
- https://www.rcog.org.uk/globalassets/documents/guidelines/scientific-impact-papers/sip_52.pdf

7. d. Biopsy of contralateral ovary

Surgery in young women is usually fertility sparing if indicated.
The main aim of surgery is to stage the disease appropriately by staging laparotomy and also to obtain tissue for diagnosis in order to aid further management. Malignant germ cell tumours are usually unilateral, although 10%–20% of the pure dysgerminomas are bilateral.
Fertility sparing surgery include the following:

- Open surgery (midline laparotomy) to aid removal of the affected ovary with its tumour rather than rupture and spill as this can lead to upstaging of the disease
- Staging of the disease (intraoperative inspection of the abdomen, pelvis, omentum and lymph nodes and excision of any visible disease)
- Unilateral oophorectomy
- Peritoneal washings
- Omental biopsy
- Selective removal of enlarged lymph nodes

Biopsy of the contralateral ovary is not indicated. Patients who underwent routine lymphadenectomy do not have a better outcome and therefore systematic lymphadenectomy is not indicated routinely in malignant ovarian germ cell tumours. Also, the presence of lymph node metastases did not have an effect on the long-term outcome. If the nodes are found to be enlarged on imaging or at laparotomy, then removal of those affected nodes is indicated.

Fertility sparing surgery did not have negative impact on survival.
For FIGO stage Ia disease, there is no need for neoadjuvant or adjuvant chemotherapy. If the disease is advanced FIGO stage Ic/II and higher, then one needs to consider administering neoadjuvant chemotherapy prior to surgery in order to help preserve fertility and decrease complexity of surgery.

In women, who do not wish to preserve fertility/completed family, completion surgery should be offered (removal of both tubes and ovaries and the uterus ((bilateral salpingo-oophorectomy and hysterectomy).

Further reading

- RCOG: Scientific Impact Paper No. 52. Management of female malignant ovarian germ cell tumours. November 2016. https://www. rcog.org.uk/globalassets/documents/guidelines/scientific-impact-papers/sip_52.pdf
- StratOG: RCOGs online learning resource. https://stratog.rcog.org.uk/ tutorial/germ-cell-tumours/presentation-4240, https://stratog.rcog.org. uk/tutorial/germ-cell-tumours/surgery-4251

8. c. Embryonal carcinoma

Malignant ovarian germ cell tumours	Tumour markers
Dysgerminoma	LDH, placental alkaline phosphatase β-hCG (low serum levels) can be raised in 3%–5% of the cases when syncytiotrophoblast multinucleated giant cells are present in dysgerminomas
Endodermal sinus tumour or yolk sac tumour	AFP is raised and LDH may be raised
Embryonal carcinomas	Both AFP and β-hCG are raised. Oestradiol can be also raised and can lead to precocious puberty
Polyembryonoma	Both AFP and β-hCG are raised
Choriocarcinoma	β-hCG is raised
Mixed germ cell tumours	Any of the above markers can be raised and depends on the components in the tumour
Immature teratoma	AFP and LDH may be raised

Raised tumour marker levels in the presence of ovarian mass helps in the initial diagnosis of malignant ovarian germ cell tumours, treatment planning, follow-up monitoring and post-treatment surveillance.

Further reading

- RCOG: Scientific Impact Paper No. 52. Management of female malignant ovarian germ cell tumours. November 2016.

9. d. Immature teratoma
- Malignant ovarian germ cell tumour.
- It occurs more commonly before 20 years of age (first two decades of life).
- It is rare after menopause.
- Second most common ovarian malignant germ cell tumour.

- Accounts for 35%–36% or one-third of the ovarian malignant germ cell tumours.
- It causes 30% of the deaths before the age of 20 years.
- It is associated with poor prognosis.

Histology

Macroscopically, they are large tumours up to 25 cm in size, predominantly solid with a capsule. Often there are areas of haemorrhage and necrosis. A mature teratoma may be present in the contralateral ovary in 10% of cases.

Microscopically, it is derived from all the three germ layers, including ectoderm, mesoderm and endoderm. Unlike mature teratomas, immature teratomas contain immature embryonic tissue. Mature elements can be present at times, but the presence of immature element confirms the diagnosis. The grading of the immature teratoma is mainly based on the quantity of immature neuroepithelial tissue as this is the most common type of tissue present in immature teratomas.

Further reading

- RCOG: Scientific Impact Paper No. 52. Management of female malignant ovarian germ cell tumours. November 2016. https://www.rcog.org.uk/globalassets/documents/guidelines/scientific-impact-papers/sip_52.pdf
- Yanai-Inbar I, Scully RE. Relation of ovarian dermoid cysts and immature teratomas: An analysis of 350 cases of immature teratoma and 10 cases of dermoid cyst with microscopic foci of immature tissue. *International Journal of Gynecologic Pathology* 1987; 6(3):203–212.
- http://pubs.rsna.org/doi/full/10.1148/rg.343130067
- https://www.rcog.org.uk/globalassets/documents/guidelines/scientific-impact-papers/sip_52.pdf
- StratOG: RCOGs online learning resource. https://stratog.rcog.org.uk/tutorial/germ-cell-tumours/tumour-markers-4239

10. d. Struma ovarii of the ovary

Struma ovarii is a histological diagnosis. In 5%–20% of the dermoid cyst, thyroid tissue may be present. However, struma ovarii is set aside when the cyst contains predominantly thyroid tissue. It can occur in pure form or as a mixture of mature cystic teratoma and thyroid tissue. Struma ovarii accounts for 2.7% of all ovarian teratomas and 0.5% of all malignant ovarian tumours (malignancy is present in 5%–10% of cases). Usually they are confined to the ovary. Mostly patients are asymptomatic and present only with pelvic mass (usually the mass is unilateral), but in 5% of the cases they can present with clinical hyperthyroidism.

The most common malignant struma ovarii is follicular carcinoma. Microscopically, it constitutes mature thyroid tissue (multiple acini filled with colloid and lined by single layer of columnar or flattened epithelium). Cellular atypia, pleomorphic nuclei, capsular invasion, vascular invasion and distant mestastasis point towards malignant struma ovarii.

Further reading

- Kostoglou-Athanassiou I, Lekka-Katsouli I, Gogou L, Papagrigoriou L, Chatonides I, Kaldrymides P. Malignant struma ovarii: Report of a case and review of the literature. *Hormone Research in Paediatrics* 2002; 58(1):34–38.

11. e.   HPV 16

HPV 16 and 18 are found in the majority of squamous cell carcinoma of the cervix. However, there are many other subtypes. Some of these cause warts and appear to be harmless, whereas others carry a risk but are less frequently found associated with malignancy.

Human papilloma virus (HPV) is a double-stranded DNA virus. It can be transmitted sexually and has a predilection to affect squamous epithelium, resulting in cellular transformation. This involves loss of maturation in the squamous epithelium (transformation to less differentiated cell type) of the cervix.

Its viral genome is made of early (E) and late (L) regions. The early region contains eight open reading frames (ORFs), which code proteins responsible for viral maintenance and replication. The late region has two ORFs, which produce proteins that form the viral capsid. Integration of the virus into the host cell DNA plays an important role in the development of cervical intraepithelial neoplasia (CIN) and cervical cancer.

HPV is present in >99% of cervical cancer. There is considerable evidence that HPV is necessary for the development of the majority of cervical cancer and its precursor lesion, CIN. HPV infection can be sexually transmitted; women carrying this virus are usually asymptomatic and the infection may be transient. However, if the HPV virus persists in the cervix, then it may lead to high-grade CIN and ultimately cervical cancer. In the United Kingdom, HPV type 16 accounts for 60%–80% of high-grade CIN and cervical cancer. The remainder of cancers is mostly caused by HPV types 18, 31, 33 and 35. HPV 6 and 11 (low-risk types) cause benign viral warts. The high-risk HPVs are types 16, 18, 31, 33, 35, 39, 45, 51, 52, 56 and 58.

Prevention of cervical cancer is the best strategy if possible. This could be achieved in two ways: (1) Taking measures to avoid the risk factors (early age of intercourse, multiple sexual partners, smoking, etc.) leading to development of CIN and cervical cancer. (2) Early detection of precancerous abnormalities of the cervix (CIN) and treatment. One way to achieve the second option is to remove the whole transformation zone (excisional form of treatment of CIN) to treat CIN and eradicate HPV. The success rate of this treatment is 95%. The latest innovation is the HPV vaccine to prevent CIN and cervical cancer.

Further reading

- http://www.cancerscreening.nhs.uk/cervical/risk-factors-cervical-cancer.html

- Sarris, I, Sangeeta A, Susan B. *Training in Obstetrics and Gynaecology: The Essential Curriculum*. Oxford, UK: Oxford University Press, 2009, pp. 394–395.

12. b.   Adenocarcinoma of cervix

CGIN stands for cervical glandular intraepithelial neoplasia. This tends to arise in the cervical canal from the glandular columnar epithelium and is less well detected on smear. The smear referral is usually reported as glandular neoplasia and this would warrant a 2-week wait referral to colposcopy. The risk of detection of cancer in such women who are referred to with a smear abnormality of glandular neoplasia is around 40%–44%.

Further reading

- Sarris I, Sangeeta A, Susan B. *Training in Obstetrics and Gynecology: The Essential Curriculum*. Oxford, UK: Oxford University Press, 2009, pp. 391–416.

13. d.   Rhabdomyosarcoma

Rhabdomyosarcoma is an aggressive malignant tumour which usually occurs in female infants and young children. It accounts for 4%–6% of all malignancy during this period.

Sarcoma botryoides is the most common type seen in this age group. It arises from embryonic muscle cells and these present as a submucosal lesions giving the appearance "grape like." Hence, this is called sarcoma botryoides. Sarcoma botryoides is often reported as vaginal tumour in infants and children less than 5 years of age. The next most common sites include vulva and uterus.

Further reading

- Sarris I, Sangeeta A, Susan B. *Training in Obstetrics and Gynecology: The Essential Curriculum*. Oxford, UK: Oxford University Press, 2009, pp. 391–416.
- Embryonal rhabdomyosarcoma: Surgical pathology of the GI tract, liver, biliary tract and pancreas (2nd ed), 2009.
- https://www.sciencedirect.com/topics/medicine-and-dentistry/embryonal-rhabdomyosarcoma

14. a.   Molar pregnancy

Molar pregnancy belongs to a group of condition called gestational trophoblastic disease (GTD).

GTD are more common in Asian women, women over 40 years of age and teenagers.

Molar pregnancy (hydatidiform mole) is an abnormal pregnancy where the gestational trophoblasts outgrow and proliferate in clusters in the uterus. These look like grapes. It occurs when a non-viable fertilized egg implants in the uterine cavity.

There are two types:

a. Partial mole (69XXY): These occur when two sperms (diandry) fertilize a normal egg and, therefore, has three set of chromosomes (it is also called triploid pregnancy). There may be some early signs of fetal development seen on ultrasound scan, but this will not progress to develop to baby.

b. Complete mole (46XX): These occur when a single sperm fertilizes an empty egg (no genetic material) and then sperm duplicates to still have a normal number of chromosomes (both sets of 23 chromosomes derived from father). This is called androgenesis. It can also occur when two sperms fertilize an empty egg.

Further reading

● Sarris I, Sangeeta A, Susan B. *Training in Obstetrics and Gynecology: The Essential Curriculum*. Oxford, UK: Oxford University Press, 2009, pp. 391–416.

● RCOG: Information for you: Published in December 2011 (next review date: 2015).

● https://www.rcog.org.uk/globalassets/documents/patients/patient-information-leaflets/pregnancy/pi-gestational-trophoblastic-disease.pdf

15. b. Meigs syndrome

Meigs syndrome is mainly caused due to ovarian fibromas. When a benign pelvis mass (such as ovarian fibroma or fibroids) is associated with ascites and right-sided pleural effusion, it is named Meigs syndrome.

Further reading

● Sarris I, Sangeeta A, Susan B. *Training in Obstetrics and Gynecology: The Essential Curriculum*. Oxford, UK: Oxford University Press, 2009, pp. 391–416.

16. c. Granulosa-theca cell tumour

Granulosa cell tumour belong to sex-cord stromal tumours in ovarian tumour classification. This tumour produces oestrogen hormone causing unopposed action of oestrogen on the endometrium and therefore leading to develop endometrial hyperplasia and endometrial cancer.

Further reading

● Sarris I, Sangeeta A, Susan B. *Training in Obstetrics and Gynecology; The Essential Curriculum*. Oxford, UK: Oxford University Press, 2009, pp. 391–416.

17. d. Endometrial carcinoma

This woman will have a condition known as Lynch syndrome. Lynch syndrome increases the risk of both colorectal cancer and endometrial cancer. Young women diagnosed with Lynch syndrome should be kept under surveillance with yearly colonoscopy and endometrial biopsy.

Ideally these women need to be referred to a genetic clinic for appropriate counselling and monitoring. These women need to be counselled thoroughly to complete their family early and should be offered combined oral contraceptive pills if not planning to conceive as this can reduce the risk of endometrial cancer by almost 50%. Once her family is complete, then she should be offered prophylactic hysterectomy.

Further reading

- Sarris I, Sangeeta A, Susan B. *Training in Obstetrics and Gynecology: The Essential Curriculum*. Oxford, UK: Oxford University Press, 2009, pp. 391–416.

18. d.   Stomach

This is called Krukenburg tumour. It occurs due to metastasis from the gastrointestinal tract tumours to the ovary. The most common primary is from stomach. The typical cells seen on histology of these metastatic GI tumours to ovaries are "signet ring" cells. These tumours on the ovary are usually bilateral and symmetrical on both sides.

Further reading

- Sarris I, Sangeeta A, Susan B. *Training in Obstetrics and Gynecology: The Essential Curriculum*. Oxford, UK: Oxford University Press, 2009, pp. 391–416.

KNOWLEDGE AREA 15: UROGYNAECOLOGY AND PELVIC FLOOR PROBLEMS

QUESTIONS

1. You are the in the urogynaecology clinic, and you are about to see a 56-year-old woman who complains of incontinence on coughing and sneezing. She also reports urgency, and she is occasionally incontinent with it. What does the history indicate?
   a. Mixed incontinence
   b. Over active bladder
   c. Overflow incontinence
   d. Pelvic organ prolapse
   e. Stress incontinence

2. In urodynamics, which of the following is false?
   a. The rectal pressure probe measures the intra-abdominal pressure
   b. The bladder pressure probe measures the intravesical pressure
   c. Free uroflowmetry measures how fast the patient can empty her bladder
   d. A cough or Valsalva manoeuvre can be performed to confirm genuine stress incontinence
   e. Cystometry alone can demonstrate the reasons for voiding difficulties

3. You are in the urogynaecology clinic, and you are about to see a 56-year-old woman who complains of urge incontinence, frequency and nocturia. She does not complain of any haematuria and has no other symptoms. What is your initial investigation?
   a. Cystoscopy
   b. Post-void residual measurement
   c. Ultrasound of the kidneys, urinary tract and bladder
   d. Urine dipstick
   e. Urodynamics

4. You are in the urogynaecology clinic, and you are seeing a patient complaining of incontinence on sneezing, coughing and jumping. She has no past medical history and is not on any regular medication. Her BMI is 28 and is otherwise fit and well. Her urine dipstick was negative. What is your advice?

a. Oxybutynin
b. Pelvic floor exercise for 3 months
c. Pelvic floor exercise for 4 months
d. Weight loss
e. Urodynamics

5. Which one of the following statements is incorrect?
   a. Contractions of the detrusor muscle is controlled by sympathetic neurones
   b. Urinary incontinence is defined as the involuntary leakage of urine
   c. The hypogastric nerve is the sympathetic innervation of the bladder
   d. The trigonal mucosa is mesodermal in origin
   e. The urethra is endodermal in origin

6. You are in the urogynaecology clinic, and you are reviewing a 60-year-old woman who was examined 4 weeks ago by your colleague. She complains of urge incontinence, nocturia and frequency. She was started on oral Oxybutynin since then, and she says it has not made any difference to her symptoms. What is your advice?
   a. Botulinum toxin A injection
   b. Botulinum toxin B injection
   c. Keep taking medication for another 4 weeks
   d. Pelvic floor exercises
   e. Change to tolterodine

7. You are in the urogynaecology clinic. You are examining a 64-year-old woman who was referred to because of recurrent urinary tract infections, requiring repeated doses of antibiotics. She feels that she has incomplete emptying of her bladder and incontinence. She has a BMI of 25 and no past medical history. She is not taking any medication. There is no pelvic organ prolapse. What is the most appropriate investigation?
   a. Blood test to assess kidney function
   b. Cystoscopy
   c. Pelvic ultrasound
   d. Urine dipstick
   e. Urodynamics

8. You are in the urogynaecology clinic. You are reviewing a 64-year-old woman who was referred to because of recurrent urinary tract infections, requiring repeated doses of antibiotics. She feels that she has incomplete emptying of her bladder and urinary retention has been confirmed. She has a BMI of 25 and no past medical history. She is not on any medication. There is no pelvic organ prolapse. What is the correct treatment?
   a. Anticholinergic drugs
   b. Bladder catheterization
   c. Botulinum toxin A
   d. Conservative management
   e. Pelvic floor exercises

ANSWERS

1. a.   Mixed incontinence

   This woman has symptoms of mixed incontinence. The treatment should be directed toward the predominant symptom, which in this case is stress incontinence.

   Further reading

   - National Institute for Health and Care Excellence. *Urinary Incontinence and Pelvic Organ Prolapse in Women: Management. NG123.* London, UK: NICE, 2019.
   - Abrams P, Cardozo L, Fall M et al. The standardization of terminology of lower urinary tract function: Report from the standardization sub-committee of the international continence society. *Neurourology and Urodynamics* 2002; 21:167–178.

2. e.   Cystometry alone can demonstrate the reasons for voiding difficulties

   Free uroflowmetry measures how fast the patient can empty his or her bladder. Multichannel cystometry measures the pressure in the rectum and in the bladder, using two separate pressure catheters, to deduce the vesical pressure and the presence of contractions of the bladder wall during bladder filling or other provocative manoeuvres. The strength of the urethra can also be tested during this phase, using a cough or Valsalva manoeuvre, to confirm genuine stress incontinence. Pressure uroflowmetry also measures the rate of voiding but with simultaneous assessment of bladder and rectal pressures. It helps demonstrate the reasons for difficulty in voiding, for example, bladder muscle weakness or obstruction of the bladder outflow.

   Further reading

   - RCOG online learning resource: StratOG: Urogynaecology and pelvic floor problems. https://elearning.rcog.org.uk/tutorials/core-training/ urogynaecology-and-pelvic-floor-problems

3. d.   Urine dipstick

   A urine dipstick should be undertaken for all women presenting with urinary incontinence to check for the presence of blood, glucose, protein, leucocytes and nitrates. If it is positive and the woman is symptomatic, then antibiotics should be given.

   Further reading

   - National Institute for Health and Care Excellence. *Urinary Incontinence and Pelvic Organ Prolapse in Women: Management. NG123.* London, UK: NICE, 2019.
   - Irwin DE, Milsom I, Hunskaar S et al. Population-based survey of urinary incontinence, overactive bladder, and other lower urinary tract symptoms in five countries: Results of the EPIC study. *European Urology* 2006; 50:1306–1314.

4. b.   Pelvic floor exercise for 3 months

A trial of supervised pelvic floor exercises should be offered as first line, for 3 months, in any patient with a history of stress incontinence.

Further reading

● National Institute for Health and Care Excellence. *Urinary Incontinence and Pelvic Organ Prolapse in Women: Management. NG123*. London, UK: NICE, 2019.
● Saleh S, Majumdar A, Williams K. The conservative (non-pharmacological) management of female urinary incontinence. *The Obstetrician & Gynaecologist* 2014; 16:169–177.

5. a.   Contractions of the detrusor muscle is controlled by sympathetic neurones

It is the parasympathetic neurones which control the contraction of the detrusor smooth muscle and the relaxation of the outflow tract.

Further reading

● RCOG online learning resource: StratOG: Urogynaecology and pelvic floor problems. https://elearning.rcog.org.uk/tutorials/core-training/urogynaecology-and-pelvic-floor-problems

6. e.   Tolterodine

If a medication does not work within 4 weeks, then NICE recommends another medication to be tried for the next 4 weeks, before botulinum toxin A injection is given.

Further reading

● National Institute for Health and Care Excellence. *Urinary Incontinence and Pelvic Organ Prolapse in Women: Management. NG123*. London, UK: NICE; 2019.

7. c.   Pelvic ultrasound

In this case, the woman has urinary retention, which causes urinary infection. Once it is confirmed, appropriate treatment will be required.

Further reading

● RCOG online learning resource: StratOG: Urogynaecology and pelvic floor problems. https://elearning.rcog.org.uk/tutorials/core-training/urogynaecology-and-pelvic-floor-problems

8. b.   Bladder catheterization

This can be either intermittent or indwelling urethral or suprapubic. It is the treatment of choice for urinary retention causing incontinence, infections or renal dysfunction.

Further reading

- National Institute for Health and Care Excellence. *Urinary Incontinence and Pelvic Organ Prolapse in Women: Management. NG123.* London, UK: NICE, 2019.
- Leydon GM, Turner S, Smith H, Little P. Women's views about management and cause of urinary tract infection: Qualitative interview study. *BMJ* 2010; 340:407.

INDEX